MANAGING PARKINSON'S

MY SIXTEEN YEAR JOURNEY

BY
VR PETERSON

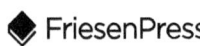 FriesenPress

One Printers Way
Altona, MB R0G 0B0
Canada

www.friesenpress.com

ISBN
978-1-03-918775-7 (Hardcover)
978-1-03-918774-0 (Paperback)
978-1-03-918776-4 (eBook)

1. Health & Fitness, Diseases, Alzheimer's & Dementia

Distributed to the trade by The Ingram Book Company

Table of Contents

The Road Not Taken

Robert Frost (1874-1963)

Two roads diverged in a yellow wood,
And sorry I could not travel both.
And be one traveler, long I stood
And looked down one as far as I could
To where it bent in the undergrowth;

Then took the other, as just as fair,
And having perhaps the better claim,
Because it was grassy and wanted wear;
Though as for that the passing there
Had worn them really about the same,

And both that morning equally lay
In leaves no step had trodden black.
Oh, I kept the first for another day!
Yet knowing how way leads on to way,

I doubted if I should ever come back.

I shall be telling this with a sigh
Somewhere ages and ages hence:
Two roads diverged in a wood, and I-
I took the one less traveled by,
And that has made all the difference.

Author's Note

A diagnosis of Parkinson's disease (PD) is a life-altering event. There is no one way to deal with it. Everyone has a unique set of circumstances, and every patient experiences the disease differently. In "Managing Parkinson's", I write as a professional educator and patient to tell my story of being diagnosed with PD for over 16 years.

My book provides the reader with a clear understanding of the disease itself. It addresses both motor and non-motor symptoms and how they affect individuals diagnosed with the disease. It offers the reader additional means to manage and cope with the progression of the disease. Topics such as nutrition, the power of exercise, and answers to frequently asked questions highlight the importance of choosing the right path in adjusting to a new and positive lifestyle.

My key players are identified and show the importance of my support team that has helped me to adjust to a new and positive lifestyle.

Another special feature is a detailed discussion between myself and my neurologist after each scheduled appointment. The findings and recommendations are outlined in the form of a timeline giving rise to my "reaction and insights." Hopefully, you will draw your own reactions and insights and find ways to successfully manage this chronic disease.

Prologue

I learned of my fate on a cold and dreary day in January 2007 when I was sixty -one years old. My family doctor expressed concern about a tremor in my right foot and soreness in my right shoulder. He referred me to the Foothills Medical Centre Movement Disorder Clinic in Calgary, Alberta. Two young student neurologists recorded my medical history and conducted a series of simple tests. They asked me to perform such tasks as: rotating my hands back-and-forth, touching my index finger and thumb together, tapping my foot up and down as quickly as I could. They tested my reflexes with a reflex hammer. They watched as I tracked a moving object with my eyes. They asked me to walk up and down the hall observing my gait and ability to make turns without losing my balance.

The Director of the Movement Clinic, who was also the teaching neurologist, came in later and performed a series of similar tests confirming a diagnosis of Parkinson's disease. She assured me that the symptoms were mild and confined to the right side of my body. I would need treatment with drugs to offset my condition.

You must be joking! I asked: "What is Parkinson's disease? Why is this happening to me? What caused this to happen? Can Parkinson's be slowed, stopped, or even reversed? I was hoping to find definitive answers. As far as I could conclude there was no evidence of Parkinson's disease in my family, both past and present. My parents lived well into their 90s with few medical issues and certainly not PD.

My neurologist described dopamine [1]as a type of neurotransmitter and hormone. It plays a role in many important body functions, including movement, memory and pleasurable reward and motivation. High or low levels of dopamine are associated with several mental health and neurological diseases. Parkinson's is a disease with gradually diminishing levels of dopamine. She prescribed amantadine, a dopamine agonist[2] which is widely used to treat mild cases of PD. She told me to observe how it worked and report back in three months, unless I experienced problems.

I was devastated with the diagnosis. Driving home was somewhat surreal. Too many unanswered questions continued to flood my mind. My entire body felt like it was being invaded by quicksand. More questions: "How would my family react to the news that I have been diagnosed with Parkinson's Disease? How might you, the reader, have reacted in similar circumstances?"

January 19, 2007, I am reminded of the original classic 1951 science fiction movie starring, Michael Rennie and Patricia Neale entitled, *"The Day the Earth Stood Still."* A day when my Earth felt a mix of confusion and disbelief. As for the prescribed dopamine agonist, the results were quite negative. I had difficulty sleeping and then waking up every two hours after having disturbing dreams. The right side of my body felt stiff and uncomfortable.

Robert Frost's poem, *"The Road Not Taken"* came to mind when considering choices or paths to follow in response to being diagnosed. One road can represent denial or refusing to believe that something is true, valid or appropriate. The other would represent acceptance or being able to look at something as it is. Accepting something does not imply judgment about it, just an honest consideration of reality. Was the diagnosis wrong? Would I continue to be in denial?

In fact, it took me more than a year to process the diagnosis. I'm still processing it. I engaged a few coping strategies to prevent being discovered. I didn't reach out to other PD patients. I kept my diagnosis to myself and my family. As you will note later in this manuscript, I did indeed select my road correctly.

My neurologist asked if I would like to take part in a research study of a new drug that did not yet have a name, but only a number: SLV308[3]. This was an investigational drug since it had not been approved by Health Canada or other health authorities for sale at that time. It was to be tested in this study to see whether it would help in treating the symptoms of

PD. About 140 people had received SLV308 so far in previous clinical studies. If I agreed to be part of the research study, I would take this experimental drug and continue taking amantadine[4] for mild cases of PD and trazodone[5] to help me sleep.

By late April 2007, I felt nauseous, tension in my back and shoulders, stiffness on my right side, and loss of energy. By mid-June 2007, I experienced a burning sensation in my stomach and esophagus. An on-call neurologist prescribed two more drugs, "Domperidone[6] for my stomach, and omeprazole[7] for chest pains." By mid-June, I was taking four different medications, plus the experimental drug, daily. My symptoms failed to improve. I experienced severe headaches, dizziness, chest pains, and stiffness in both hands. At one point, I collapsed on the floor and had difficulty getting up.

By late June 2007, I asked to be withdrawn from the research study. Was this the right decision? You can read more about this study in Part 7, "Your Role in Clinical Trials." In its place, my neurologist prescribed Apo-Levocarb 100/25mg[8] taken three times daily with meals. In the months that followed, I was frightened about my future and illness. As part of the study, she asked that I meet with Dr. Quickfall, a resident Psychiatrist.

During July and August 2007, my condition improved, and I began to think more clearly. I was less in denial and more focused in changing my lifestyle. I asked myself more questions: "Does my family know anything about this chronic disease? Would participating in research help in my own understanding in how to cope with a changing lifestyle? Where would I find accurate information about Parkinson's disease? Would this knowledge assist others that may find themselves in a similar scenario about PD? Should I write a self-help manuscript to assist others diagnosed with PD? Would the manuscript be useful for my own family, medical support team, close friends, and others that may be inflicted with this chronic disease? How could I design and write the manuscript in a unique way that others would find useful? Or was I still in denial? Which road would I choose from Robert Frost's *The Road Not Taken?*"

An important feature of this manuscript is a discussion between my neurologist and me. Every six months, I met and was examined by my neurologist. The highlights of her report are stated in point form. My reactions and insights are revealed in the response.

A more detailed timeline of the neurologist and patient's report is found in Appendix 1. For example,

June 15, 2007, the neurologist, Dr. Suchowersky reported:
- The Titration Research Study has been closed due to several issues and concerns.
- The patient's negative reactions were probably the result of taking a much higher strength dosage of the experimental drug.
- No conclusive findings were evident from the study.
- The drug "Apo-Levocarb 100/25mg" would continue to be prescribed for the patient to be taken three times daily (breakfast, lunch, and dinner) to alleviate Parkinson's symptoms.
- The patient would see the resident Psychiatrist, Dr. Quickfall, as part of the research study.

June 22, 2007, Dr. Quickfall, Psychiatrist summed up the meeting:
- The patient's anxiety was mostly due to his illness.
- The patient's presented himself to be very intelligent and articulate man.
- He articulated lots of insights into his own condition and various ways to address them.
- His form was linear, and goal protected.
- He had no obvious perceptual or cognitive impairments.
- Recommended dealing with anxiety with non-pharmacological means as much as possible.
- To help control his symptoms, suggested reading the *"Anxiety & Phobia Workbook,"* by Edmund Bourne, Ph.D.
- Prescribed a low strength medication, Pms-Clonazepam 0.5mg[9] taken once daily when needed to control his anxiety.
- Suggested a follow-up visit after two months.

Follow-up visit, August 27, 2007, Dr. Quickfall, Psychiatrist reported:
- Patient's anxiety has remarkably improved over the summer months.

- He showed a positive adjustment to his Parkinson's diagnosis.
- The drug trazodone taken nightly helped his sleep cycle.
- No underlying acute anxiety disorder requiring further treatment is needed.

VR's Reaction and Insights

I was pleased that my neurologist recommended Levo-Carb (Sinemet)[10] to control my PD symptoms. Over the summer months, my condition improved immensely. I was somewhat apprehensive about having to see a psychiatrist, but Dr. Quickfall's assessment and recommendations were very helpful easing my anxiety.

Was I still in denial? Probably, because there were so many questions to be asked and so few answers. Based on my experience, I would not recommend taking part in a research study during the initial phase of being diagnosed. Would I continue to be involved in research studies at a later stage? Definitely, to "pay it forward" supporting others in a quest to find a cure or means to slow down the progression of the disease. Overall, my acceptance and willingness to adapt to a new lifestyle was about to begin.

I must acknowledge beloved Canadian actor Michael J. Fox, who was recognized with one of Hollywood's biggest honours for his advocacy since he was diagnosed with Parkinson's disease. For raising $1.5 billion for Parkinson's research, the "*Back to the Future* and *Family Ties*" star was awarded an Oscar statuette: the Jean Hersholt Humanitarian Award.

Michael J. Fox was just 29 years old when diagnosed with Parkinson's disease. He remained in denial for 7 years while trying to make sense of the disease. Now at 61 years of age, Fox remains committed to finding a means of slowing down the progression of PD or finding a cure.

PART 1 -
What Is Parkinson's Disease?

Part 1 addresses many basic questions, giving the reader an understanding and insight into Parkinson's disease. It explains the disease and from different sources of research addresses causes, diagnosis, and prognosis.

Parkinson's disease is a common illness of the nervous system. It affects the functioning of a small part of the brain called the "substantia nigra"[11] As this part of the brain degenerates, a chemical in the brain called "dopamine" is lost. Dopamine helps transmit signals or messages from the brain to different parts of the body. This occurs when dopamine levels are reduced by about 80 percent. As such, it is a chronic disease that gets worse over time. The good news is that the disease progresses slowly and takes years before it affects a person's quality of life.

What Causes Parkinson's Disease?

Apparently, there is no conclusive answer to this question. There are numerous theories and possible causes, none have yet to be proven. The name comes from Dr. James Parkinson, who first described it in 1817.

Age is clearly the most important risk factor. Estimates indicate that over 10 million people worldwide have the disease. In Canada alone, the number is about 100,000 people. 1 in 100 over the age of 65 develop the disease. Men are more likely than women to develop Parkinson's disease. As we age, all of us lose dopamine producing nerve cells which results in the slower, more measured movements. Those diagnosed with Parkinson's lose their dopamine faster.

Genetics might play a significant role, but research suggests otherwise. In fact, only about 10% of Parkinson's disease can be linked to a genetic cause.

Head Injuries are four times more likely to develop Parkinson's than those who have never suffered a head injury. Researchers caution us that this does not mean head injuries cause PD.

Environmental (exposure to metals) or industrial toxic chemicals (pesticides and herbicide) may play a role in increasing the risk of developing Parkinson's disease.

How Do We Know It Is Parkinson's Disease?

No single diagnostic test can confirm a clinical diagnosis of Parkinson's Disease. During my first examination I was asked several questions about my medical history. Following that the neurologist measured blood pressure with me lying down and standing up. The final evaluation was an examination through a process of observation. The neurologist tested my coordination and balance while I walked, stood, sat and turned around. Other tasks included: opening and closing my fists or tapping my fingers several times; touching my neurologist's finger then my nose with my index finger; recovering my balance after she pulled me gently from behind my shoulders as I stood with my eyes opened then closed. I answered several simple questions to test my attention and memory. I drew a figure on a piece of paper and duplicated it. The neurologist used a standardized rating scale to measure symptoms and stages of the disease.

Though Parkinson's disease is traditionally thought of as a disease that only older people get, there are many younger people living with the disease as well. The average age of diagnosis for Parkinson's is early 60s. When seen in individuals under the age of 40, it is called "younger or early onset" PD. About 10% of the total population with Parkinson's will be diagnosed as early onset PD. In this case, there is often genetic factors at play.

Parkinson's Prognosis

Do people die from Parkinson's? No, people die with Parkinson's. They may have died from other causes as these become more common in advanced stages.

How fast does PD progress? It varies from one person to another. For me the disease remained static for the first ten years. In some cases, severe disability can occur within a few years. Most people will have a progression that falls somewhere between these two extremes. Those people whose first symptoms were basically a tremor have experienced a slower progression in the disease. It is important to note that everybody is different, and symptoms may progress differently for each of us.

Is it possible to slow down the progression of PD? Scientists have not been able to find a way to change the ultimate course of the disease. Early treatment has been shown to delay disease progression. Vitamins C, E, and selenium have been linked to possibly helping slow the progression of the disease.

VR's Reaction and Insights

Here are some of the questions I asked after being diagnosed, to which I received no definitive answers:

- **"Why me?"** Again, limited response as there was no history of Parkinson's in my family.
- **"What causes PD?"** One theory suggests some toxin in the environment triggered a gene that resulted in the loss of "dopamine" in an area of the brain.
- **"Is it hereditary?"** Again, a limited response suggesting that it is probably more the environment.
- **"Is there any margin of error in the neurologist's diagnosis?"** I must admit that looking at the various stages of progression enhances one's fear of the consequences. I was surprised that my neurologist performed such simple physical tests in diagnosing the disease.

- **"Has the diagnosis raised my level of anxiety?"** It's not a death sentence, but definitely there is a need to make significant changes in one's life style.
- **"Am I in denial?"** You bet, and it lasted for over a year. On dealing with life's challenges, I've always set goals for myself in a positive manner. I couldn't accept defeat, so I focused on learning more about the disease.

PD patients meet with their neurologist every six months for examinations. I was involved in a research study, and I met with my neurologist every three months. I talked with her honestly about my symptoms I was experiencing. This would help her recommend the best possible medications, so I could remain independent.

Parkinson's is a disease that is constantly changing. It is chronic (lasting many years) and progressive (worsens over time). As there is currently no cure for Parkinson's, the goal is to keep it in check.

PART 2 -
Parkinson's Motor Symptoms

Part 2 describes each of the motor symptoms stressing there is no "one-size-fits" all. Most people with PD live a full and productive life for many years. "Helpful suggestions" are included after each "motor symptom" described.

Resting Tremor

In the early stages of the disease, I experienced a slight tremor in the hand and foot on my right side. Because tremor usually appears when the muscles are relaxed, it's called a "resting tremor." Tremors can temporarily worsen during periods of anxiety, stress, and fatigue. I had found that my tremors were more of an annoyance than a disability.

Helpful Suggestions

Research studies has suggested caffeine may be able to help control tremors. Drinking small amounts of alcohol may reduce tremor. However, I have found that too much alcohol can make tremors worse. There is also a surgical procedure called "deep brain stimulation" that can be used to treat tremors. Deep brain stimulation[12] is used only for people in the latter stage of development.

Rigidity

Rigidity or stiffness refers to a lack of flexibility in the muscles of your arms, legs, body or neck. Rigidity can result in a decreased range of motion. Rigidity can also cause pain and cramps at the muscle site.

Helpful Suggestions

I do my stretching exercises and walking three or four times a week at our local YMCA which has kept me quite limber. I also go for a massage every two weeks. I thoroughly enjoy the pushing and prodding done by my therapist.

Bradykinesia (Slow Movement)

Bradykinesia refers to movements becoming slower and smaller. These movements are related to the lowering levels of dopamine in your system. I am very fortunate as this has not happened to me yet. I am still able to walk, talk, brush my teeth and cut my food. My handwriting has become smaller, but I am able to use my computer.

Helpful Suggestions

Stay active and keep a regular exercise routine. Always be open to exploring new ways to cope. Bradykinesia is very well managed with treatment, such as dopamine medication and exercise. This will help you maintain a full and productive life.

Balance Problems

This motor symptom refers to being unstable when standing upright. Difficulty with balance often occurs when you are changing position.

Helpful Suggestions

Balance training is the most important treatment for balance problems. This might include Tai chi; yoga, dance; strength-building exercises of your trunk (or torso) muscles; and aerobic exercises (bicycling, swimming, water aerobics). I try to work balance into my daily exercise program through lifting weights and standing on one foot.

VR's Reaction and Insights

The motor symptoms listed above, play a significant role in dealing with PD. During my early stages, both resting tremor and rrigidity were the most noticeable symptoms and were definitely annoying. Being tired or stressed makes matters worse. Personally, a glass of wine does help relax the body and calm both symptoms, but too much alcohol can cause negative results.

Rigidity affects my right side, especially the arm, leg, and neck area. My motor symptoms are easily controlled by medication. I found exercise can do wonders easing these symptoms. I can use a stationary bike with no difficulty but my lack of range of motion, due to recent knee replacement surgery, makes biking outside somewhat difficult. Skiing and playing golf are sports that I enjoy and partake in seasonally. As my PD has progressed, I've noticed less power in playing golf and more difficulty making right turns in skiing. I can always turn left.

My neurologist offered another research study that I thought sounded encouraging. It involved creatine, not the use of drugs. It is a chemical found naturally in the body. It's also in red meat and seafood and is often used to improve exercise performance and muscle mass. I agreed to take part because I feel it was helpful for finding a cure or method to slow down the progression of PD. A detailed explanation of the study is found in Part 7 entitled, "Your Role In Clinical Trials."

In summary, I found little difficulty with motor symptoms for approximately the first ten years. The symptoms tend to cause issues when feeling tired, experiencing anxiety, or during medication off-times. More about these challenges later. I strongly suggest keeping a diary of the symptoms you encounter and later discuss them with your doctor or neurologist.

May 19, 2010, Dr. Suchowersky reported:

- The patient is experiencing mild Parkinson's disease symptoms which are reasonably controlled with medication.
- Continue taking "Apo-Levocarb 100/25mg" three times daily with meals and "Apo-Levocarb CR 100/25mg" x1 a slow-release tablet at bedtime.
- Vic has agreed to take part in a Double-Blinded Placebo Control Trial [13] using creatine in hopes to slow down progression of Parkinson's Disease.

PART 3 -
Parkinson's Non-Motor Symptoms

Part 3 provides information about non-motor symptoms affecting PD. It enables the reader to have with help in identifying symptoms. Strategies and treatments are suggested as a means of controlling each symptom. The list is long and somewhat discouraging. In fact, there are over 20 non-motor symptoms. Remember that many of these symptoms will never happen to you personally. Most of them can be controlled with medications. I've also broken down "sleep issues" into sub-categories for more clarity.

Sleep Issues

Dyskinesia (Mobility) and Sleep Issues

Dyskinesia[14] refers to abnormal, involuntary movements. It is the result of a complex interaction in the brain between PD progression and continued use of dopamine medication. The symptoms are often worse at night. I found that I could fall asleep quickly, but then I would wake up too early and not be able to get back to sleep.

REM or Sleep Disorder

REM is another issue that affects sleep. REM or (rapid eye-movement) sleep is one of five sleep stages. Most dreaming takes place during REM sleep. Normally, your body is incapable of movement during REM sleep. This is a good thing, as it keeps you from acting out your dreams.

Daytime Sleepiness

Daytime sleepiness refers to feeling sleepy or sleeping too much during the day. If you have mild sleepiness, you may fall asleep when you are inactive.

Restless Leg Syndrome (RLS)

RLS refers to the urge to move your legs in order to try to stop an uncomfortable feeling. Typically, RLS happens when you are sitting or lying down. It tends to be worse in the evening and at night. For this reason, you may have trouble falling asleep.

Helpful Suggestions

There are many ways that may improve insomnia. This is a very difficult symptom to overcome. I try to not watch the clock, and I listen to music on my iPad. I exercise daily either at home or at the YMCA and I love to soak up bright sunlight in the late afternoon. I have decaffeinated tea or coffee after dinner or water. There are medical options that your doctor will help you with if you still are having trouble.

Most dreaming takes place during REM sleep. REM sleep disorder may cause you to act out your dreams. It has happened to me but very rarely. I have shouted and talked out as I relive some earlier event in my life. Melatonin[15] is the naturally available over-the-counter drug to use at bedtime. I have tried it but wasn't successful. Doctor prescribed Pms-Clonazepam (also called Rivotril) can make a big difference in improving

REM sleep. Caution must be exercised as sleeping pills have many side effects. I have a prescription and use it upon occasion.

For mild daytime sleepiness make certain that you are getting enough light exposure during the day (walk outside if you can). As I age, I find that I fall asleep more often when I and not physically active. Watching TV or listening to conversations often find me sleeping. Talk to your doctor for possible solutions.

When in bed, if I have Restless Leg Syndrome, I try walking around the room or reading for a while. I generally avoid caffeine and alcohol prior to bedtime.

VR's Reaction and Insights

I've broken down non-motor symptoms into subcategories. If you are a Person with Parkinson's (PWP) don't be discouraged because many of these symptoms, you may not experience. The symptoms that affect me the most are sleep problems. Taking any form of medications will disrupts my sleep patterns. I have no problem falling asleep but wake up every night around 3:30 - 5:00 AM. I visit the bathroom only twice during the night. Sometimes I take an extra levo-carb pill or one suggested by my neurologist as mild clonazepam 0.5 mg. I can easily tell that medications have worn off because my lower back and right leg are very stiff. During this stage, I find it difficult to turn over in bed. I experience many dreams that in most cases fail to make sense. My movements are very slow making it to the bathroom. These symptoms have worsened over time. As I awaken most mornings at around 6:00 AM I limber up and go downstairs to feed our noisy cat. My body tends to loosen up as I become more mobile.

Bodily Function Problems

Constipation

Constipation is defined as having less than three bowel movements a week, or bowel movements that are very difficult to pass. This problem affects about three or four people with PD. They can be painful, and you may need to strain. You may not feel that you can completely relax the muscles that hold in bowel movements. It happens when the nerve cells that control bowel movements in your gut die. This slows down how food matter passes through your bowels.

Bladder issues

Bladder issues affect about one out of three people with Parkinson's. The most common problem is an over-active (hyperactive) bladder which can cause you to rush to the bathroom, urinate very often, and get up several times at night. The bladder muscles are controlled by the brain and those brain centers can be affected in PD. Men who have prostate problems also need to urinate very often. The urine stream is slow and hesitant. If the stream is not slow, the prostate is usually not the cause.

Helpful Suggestions

Because constipation and bowel movement cause annoying problems, I try to drink lots of water, at least five or six glasses per day. I also try to eat foods that are rich in fibre. Moderate exercises such as walking, swimming, and gardening also help keep things moving. I find that over-the-counter products work to some degree. I go to the washroom at regular times during the day. When traveling I take note of the closest washroom especially in a new environment. If you are experiencing any of these problems tell your doctor. Although a nuisance for PWP, urinary and bowel issues are often treatable even as PD progresses.

Changes in Sex Life

Changes are common and can affect one out of two people with PD. Changes can range from a lower (hypo) or sometimes higher (hyper) sex drive. The relationship you may have enjoyed with your partner for years, suddenly comes under question. Can I adequately satisfy the needs of this person I love? Is this person trying to protect me by pretending that nothing's changed?

Another sexual problem PD patients often has to do with arousal. For men, erection issues are a common problem. As men age, PD may have a negative impact of the central nervous system, circulation, or muscle function. Men find it difficult to obtain or maintain an erection. Women might have less interest in sex due to anxiety or stress, which may eventually lead to depression.

Do men and women over 60 lose their sex drive? Do they find it difficult to have intimate relationships ending in intercourse? Many men and women find their sex life improves with age. If this isn't the case, one should talk with your doctor as some of the symptoms may be treatable.

Helpful Suggestions

For men, your doctor may suggest medications like Viagra or Cialis for erection problems. For women, your doctor might suggest medication to help with sex the drive. Though it may be less romantic, you may need to do a little planning before being intimate. Fore play is important to help with arousal.

Leg Swelling

This Is a common problem for people with PD. The lower leg seems to "fill with water." Fortunately, I have not had any leg swelling. Many non-Parkinson medications or other health problems may cause leg swelling.

Helpful Suggestions

Wear compression (or support) stockings to help the blood from pooling in your legs. Using a pillow while sit with your legs raised. See your doctor for treatment advice.

VR's Reaction and Insights

While constipation does not appear to be a major issue with me, the more water I drink increases the frequency of my trips to the bathroom during daytime. The bladder muscles are controlled by the brain and those brain centres can be affected with PD. I try to avoid large quantities of liquid and caffeine before bedtime. However, not all issues are the result of PD, but getting older may be the culprit. Other symptoms such as feeling faint, changes in sexuality, and leg swelling have not caused me any concerns so far.

Mental Ability / Health Issues

Mental Ability

Some people may have trouble with attention, thinking and memory. While somewhat bothersome, mild cognitive impairment does not typically have any serious effect on your day-to-day life. Keep in mind that forgetting sometimes is normal as we age.

Mood/Anxiety and Apathy

Mood and anxiety problems affect one out of three PWP. If you are depressed, you may not be able to experience joy. If you have anxiety, you may find yourself worrying about everyday things, even things that you should not feel anxious about. Apathy is the feeling of no interest or indifference to things or life in general. You may not be interested in doing new things. Panic attacks and anxiety can also happen during "off periods." When your medications wear off, the muscles in your chest wall can tighten.

Side Effects/Depression

Depression is very common in people with PD because of the side effects of drugs. If you experience five or more of the following symptoms for longer than two weeks at a time, you should consult your doctor. These symptoms include depressed mood, inability to find pleasure in things that were once pleasurable, sleep disturbance, change of appetite, fatigue, altered level of activity, difficulty concentrating, low self-esteem, and thoughts of death.

Helpful Suggestions

Depression can be treated with therapy, as well with drug treatments. Staying connected with friends and family, as well as exercising, can also help. Your doctor may suggest anti-depression medications or adjust your dopamine medications. Speak with your doctor or neurologist if you are having problems.

Hallucinations, Delusions

People with PD may experience hallucinations (visual, auditory, tactile) when you think something is present when it isn't or delusions (paranoia, jealousy, extravagance). A delusion is when you are convinced something is true, despite clear evidence proving that it is not. These are more apparent with those that have had the PD for a long time. I have very occasionally seen an inanimate object (a spot on the wall or floor) that appears to move or looks like something else.

Helpful Suggestions

Your doctor can check for possible causes such as an imbalance of chemicals in your blood, improper kidney, liver, or lung function, as well as certain infections. Other over-the-counter medications may be the culprit. It is a delicate balance trying to keep dyskinesia to a minimum while not hallucinating.

Stress

It is normal for someone with PD to experience anxiety. Anxiety may be a reaction to PD or it may be part of PD, related to a loss of dopamine, non-adrenalin (motivates the brain for actions), and serotonin[16] (neurotransmitter) nerve cells. Anxiety often accompanies the "off" periods when a person with PD experiences immobility. Finding the source of anxiety is the key to its lessening and possible treatment. In more severe cases, some PD persons may experience panic attacks. You may feel things like shortness of breath, clammy sweat, irregular heartbeat, dizziness, faintness, and feelings of unreality. Unfortunately, very little research has been done to figure out the best course of treatment for those who have panic attacks. Your doctor can prescribe various drugs to control the attacks.

Stress can have a very negative impact on the symptoms of Parkinson's Disease. Stress comes from a variety of different sources that can be physical, as well as emotional. Stress can come from daily life tasks, events, problems, fatigue, as well as anxiety and frustration. The important thing to be aware of is that stress can worsen PD symptoms, especially tremor and mobility. It is important to focus on stress management and relaxation in your daily life.

Helpful Suggestions

There are many ways to avoid stress that may or may not work for a person with PD. Some examples that I have tried include meditation, breathing exercises progressive relaxation (getting in a comfortable position with eyes closed) massage and mindfulness, in the form of Books/Tapes/DVDs/Podcasts. The ones that work best for me are massage and relaxation by falling asleep.

VR's Reaction and Insights

Mental issues do not appear worrisome currently, despite dealing with PD for over 16 years. Mild cognitive impairment does not typically have any serious effect on my day-to-day life. I am forever losing my glasses but have been doing so for many years. This is more a product of age. Mood, anxiety and apathy are only minor issues that cause concern. My daily activities have remained much the same. Trouble controlling impulses like excessive gambling, binge eating, compulsive shopping are not issues of concern. I will admit that there are times I have carried out pointless tasks such as sorting and re-sorting items or projects.

Mixed Motor/Non-Motor Changes

Feeling Faint

Some people may feel suddenly faint when they stand up. This faintness is caused by a drop in blood pressure. Falling blood pressure is part of the disease process. A sudden drop in blood pressure can cause dizziness, light-headedness, confusion, headache, shoulder and neck pain.

Helpful Suggestions

You can manage blood pressure drops using a variety of methods. Avoid standing up quickly. Raise the head of your bed when you sleep by putting a book or blocks under the legs of the bed. Drink plenty of water to make sure you are well hydrated and watch what you eat. Be sure you are taking enough salt in your meals. Avoid heavy meals as they can lead to a blood pressure drop. Wear compression (or support) stockings to help stopping blood from pooling in your legs.

Behaviour

In some cases, a person with PD may change his/her behaviour in certain situations. You may lack the confidence in performing tasks that you have normally done, so you avoid doing them. Self-esteem can also be greatly affected by Parkinson's. You may find it difficult being in public as the PD symptoms increase. You might feel that everyone is looking at you as you walk so you choose not to go out. However, not everyone with PD notices changes in his or her cognitive abilities.

Vision

Another significant problem or problems that you may encounter as a result of PD are blurred vision, difficulty focusing, reading, double vision, and dry eyes. Many of these conditions are frequently a part of the aging process and have easy solutions.

Helpful Suggestions

Double vision is when you see two of the same things. In PD, this is usually caused by under-active eye muscles. Speak to your optometrist if you notice this problem. Double vision can also be controlled by special lenses (prisms).

Pain

Pain affects one in three people with PD. You may have other health problems that cause you pain such as arthritis or lower back pain.

Helpful Suggestions

Practice stretching exercises to avoid pain. Schedule a massage or take a warm bath. I love to get into our hot tub in the morning and in the evening. The hot water eases my muscles. If these do not help, speak to your doctor about over-the-counter pain medications.

Drooling

Drooling refers to the buildup of saliva, which tends to leak out. Drooling happens because your mouth is moving less. It happens in about 50% of people with PD. Drooling is generally more bothersome than dangerous. For me it mostly occurs at night.

Helpful Suggestions

Chewing gum or sucking on a hard candy can help. This is because keeping something in your mouth gives you an unconscious reminder to swallow.

VR's Reaction and Insights

There are times when I feel dizzy after taking my prescribed medication. I would describe this as feeling light headedness. I also experience left shoulder and neck soreness, but I doubt this is caused by sudden low blood pressure. Could it be nerve cells in specific areas of the body not working properly?

Is my personality affected? Will it affect my behaviour? Experiencing a chronic disease must cause some changes to take place. Personally, I doubt that my behaviour has changed a great deal. I may lack some confidence in my ability to perform various certain tasks, but I still try.

For years, I wore contact lenses. At 65 years of age, I had two cataracts removed and lenses put in place. My distance vision is excellent as I no longer where glasses. I use mild strength reading glasses for close-up vision. My problem with them is that I have four pairs and can never seem to locate them. I think that's another issue. Occasionally, I do experience double vision late at night watching television. I understand this problem can be solved by special lenses (prisms) or shutting off the TV and going to bed.

Pain affects many people with PD. It may or may not have do to with Parkinson's. Like most people, as we age, arthritis, muscle pain, stiffness or lower back pain are quite common. Over the counter medications are often very helpful.

Other Non-Motor Changes

Taste and Smell

Almost all people with PD will have changes in the ability to smell, and one out of three will have no sense of smell at all. You may also notice changes in taste, as your sense of smell is directly linked to taste. This problem is not dangerous. Currently, there is no treatment available for this problem. Since the beginning I've lost my sense of smell, but not taste.

Helpful Suggestions

Since you may not be able to smell some dangerous odours, be sure that your smoke detectors are installed and are always in good working order.

Speech

It is estimated that 90% of people with PD develop speech and voice disorders. This may result in slurring of words, soft and quiet voice, and other issues. When I am tired, my speech is somewhat quieter.

Helpful Suggestions

It may be difficult to talk over television or radio. Try to carry on conversations in a quieter area. Over-articulate your speech and take time to rest your voice. It can be tiring to try to talk over the television or radio. Talk slowly and be sure the person that you were talking with can see your face. Choose a comfortable posture and position that gives you support during long and stressful conversations. Finally, plan periods of rest for your voice.

Effect on Skin

Problems occur because the autonomic nervous system is not functioning properly. It is evident for the skin on your face to become very oily, especially on your forehead and on the sides of your nose (this is known as seborrhea). You may also notice your eyebrows and scalp get oily, too, resulting in flaky skin (dandruff). It's common to experience itching, redness, and chronically inflamed areas on your skin. For years I've been dealing with psoriasis, a skin disease that causes a rash with itchy, scaly patches and in my cases is confined to my scalp. I see a dermatologist for this condition. I've also noticed some dryness on my hands. Creams and lotions help with this.

Helpful Suggestions

To help with dandruff, try an over-the-counter shampoo that has selenium, selenium sulphide, salicylic acid, zinc or coal tar in it. If your dandruff is severe, your doctor may prescribe different shampoos or lotions. Use a neutral soap like unscented glycerin soap, and always wash with warm water and rinse with cold water. Dry skin can also be a problem with PD patients. Use moisturizers and conditioners to help. I've tried many different lotions, some over the counter and others prescribed by my dermatologist. Both work for limited amounts of time. Keep trying.

Handwriting

Micrographia is characterized by writing that starts out normal size but becomes increasingly smaller and more cramped. The symptoms may appear early in the progression of your PD, later, or not at all. When medications are managing symptoms well, handwriting is normal. But as medications wear off and you get closer to the next dose, your fine motor skills may be compromised. When this happens, your writing may start strong and normal but quickly trail off into small, cramped letters, and words. When my medication is not working and I'm tired, my writing becomes much smaller. My typing has been less effective and in response I tend to use oral dictation feature on my computer.

Helpful Suggestions

I have used a computer and word processor for my written communication. Most computers have a way to dictate notes and I only must do a minimum of correction. I've have used this quite often. I also have used lined paper to help my writing stay in line.

Effect on Blood Pressure

PD persons may experience a condition called orthostatic hypotension. This is a sharp drop in blood pressure that happens when a person gets up from bed, or from a chair, which can cause light-headedness, dizziness, weakness or fainting. This is common during mid or late stages of PD. Certain prescribed medications can cause this to occur. If you feel dizzy when you stand up, but the feeling passes quickly, you probably don't have the condition. I currently don't have any issues with blood pressure. On occasion, I might feel lightheaded when I am in an off period. After workouts, my resting pulse is constant at 60 bpm. My blood pressure it's usually 80/120.

Helpful Suggestions

To prevent light headedness, I try to avoid standing for long lengths of timed I try to drink two-eight-ounce glasses of cold water to increase blood pressure. Avoid hot baths or showers, get up slowly from a lying position. Talk with your doctor about meds that may lower your blood pressure. Eat small frequent meals and try to avoid meals high in carbohydrates, especially refined carbs and sugars. Exercise gently and regularly.

Weight Loss

Change in weight is very common for PWP. Weight loss is more common than weight gain even though we tend to eat more. It is still not understood the exact reasons for Parkinson's weight changes.

Helpful Suggestions

Recently, I've noticed a slight drop in my weight. I try to take my meals during my "on" times when my medication is working well although this is not always possible. I tend to eat more during these times. High calorie foods even sweets are a good way to boost my caloric intake. I've tried liquid diet protein supplements and they are a good choice when I am going to be missing a meal or when I am doing a calorie burning activity such as golf.

Controlling Impulses

Controlling impulses affects one in eight people who are taking certain PD medications called dopamine agonists. Trouble controlling impulses is called impulsive, uncontrolled behaviour. You might have problems with excessive gambling, hyper sexuality, binge eating, compulsive shopping, and carrying out pointless tasks repeatedly. A good example may be one who sorts and resorts different items. I don't appear to have any controlling impulses. However, I do sort and resort different items.

My understanding suggests the dopamine agonist (pramipexole) is the culprit.

Helpful Suggestions

To treat this problem, your doctor will likely lower the strength of your medications.

PART 4 -
Managing With Medications

Part 4 looks at the most common medications for managing both motor and non-motor PD symptoms.

Levodopa was introduced in the 1960s and remains the most effective therapy for motor symptoms. The combination of levodopa and carbidopa (under the brand name Sinemet) is still the preferred treatment for most people with PD. Parkinson's is a disease that is constantly changing. It is chronic (lasting many years) and progressive (worsens over time). With no cure to date, the goal is to keep your symptoms in check.

As in my case, coupled with **carbidopa**, levodopa has controlled PD symptoms so far. Carbidopa's main purpose is to offset the serious and uncomfortable side effects of levodopa. The prescription includes two numbers, usually 100/25mg. The first number refers to the amount of levodopa and the second is the amount of carbidopa. This prescription is usually taken at regular intervals three to four times a day. It has a wearing-off period of about four hours. As the symptoms of PD progress your neurologist may increase the dosage and/or shorten the periods between doses. Two alternative medications are the controlled-release (CR) form of Sinemet, and orally disintegration tablet (ODT) form which prolongs the effect of levodopa.

Dopamine Agonists (DA) are drugs that imitate what levodopa does in the brain. They are often prescribed to treat PD in the early stages but can also be used in combination with carbidopa/levodopa in the later stage. My neurologist prescribed pramipexole (Mirapex). Dopamine agonists have been in use for two decades with proven effectiveness in treating PD symptoms. However, their use may be limited by troubling side effects.

One new method which might help is called a transdermal (skin) patch. The advantage of the patch is its consistent delivery of medication throughout the day. Clinical studies have shown using the patch reduces "off time." The Neupro patch, first approved for treatment in 2007 was taken off the market in 2008 because of a manufacturing issue. It has been recently approved by FDA or US Food and Drug Administration and Health Canada.

What Is the Best Way to Take My Medication?

Levodopa is best taken on an empty stomach before your meal. High protein meals can limit how much of this medication is absorbed in your stomach. So, forget that eight-ounce steak you enjoyed so much. Just remember to take your pills before the food. If you miss a dose, simply take your levodopa as soon as you remember.

My neurologist started me on a low dose of levo-carb (two pills, taken three times daily). As my condition progressed, my neurologist has increased my dosage to two pills, five times daily. There is no clear maximum dose.

I would be remiss if I failed to mention the terms "wearing off" and "on-off." The wearing-off may appear when the PWP has been on the same dosage for some time. Over time, the positive effect of the medication simply wears off before the next dose is due. In this window, the PWP may experience heightened symptoms of PD. The usual solution is to shorten the time between doses, increase strength of the medication or introduce a new medication.

The "on and off" phenomenon which is (unique to PD) refers to the PWP's ability to perform common physical activities one minute and then to be totally in capable the next minute, all within the same dosing cycle. In this case, the wearing-off effect loses its predictability, so PD symptoms emerge without warning. Track your on-off fluctuations after they begin and report your findings to your doctor or neurologist.

Report the following findings to your neurologist: the times the meds start to wear off in relation to your next scheduled dose of medicine; The exact symptoms that reappear; and the frequency if the off period.

VR's Reaction and Insights

Throughout my journey dealing with PD, I have raised more questions: "Why have they not found a cure for PD? Is there no means to slow the progression of PD?" Much of the research indicates there are no conclusive answers to these questions.

Often, I become absorbed in my daily schedule and forget to take my meds at suggested times even though I have a very loud pill timer. During so-called, "Off-Time", my symptoms tend to be more noticeable. High-protein meals can limit how much of the medication is absorbed in your stomach. It is best absorbed on empty stomach before your meal, ideally 15 to 30 minutes ahead. Make certain the pills are taken before the food. Also, try to take the meds with about five ounces of water so they can be absorbed into your body quicker. If you miss a dose, simply take your levodopa as soon as you remember.

October 26, 2011, Dr. Suchowersky reassured:
- The patient is doing well with respect to PD. There is minimal progression of symptoms over the last four years.
- He should continue taking "Apo-Levocarb 100/25mg" along with breakfast, lunch and dinner, slow release "Apo-Levocarb CR 100/25mg" at bedtime and an "Auro-Pramipexole 0.75 mg[17]" with meals.

VR's Reaction and Insights

As of April 2012, I noticed an increase in resting tremor when trying to sleep. I also reported rigidity or tightness of muscles in my right hand/arm and lower back. Again, sleep disturbance has been an issue since being diagnosed. I have no trouble falling asleep but wake up about 3 o'clock experiencing a tremor and stiffness in my trunk area.

November 7, 2012, Dr. Suchowersky reported:
- Vic experienced no side effects taking "creatine case study" for the last five years as part of a second research study.
- His condition is stable with respect to Parkinson's disease.
- No gait or balance issues.
- Continue taking "Apo-Levocarb 100/25mg" along with breakfast, lunch and dinner, slow release "Apo-Levocarb CR 100/25mg" at bedtime and an "Auro-Pramipexole 0.75 mg" with meals.

VR's Reaction and Insights

As of May 2013, I noticed an increase in tremor on my right side. This occurred mostly in early morning or late evening. There was no evidence of bradykinesia, impaired balance, or cognitive issues. Having a restful sleep remains as a challenge.

October,11, 2013, Dr. Suchowersky reported:
- Progression was minimal over the last six years.
- Medication shows very little change taking patient should continue taking "Apo-Levocarb 100/25mg" along with breakfast, lunch and dinner, slow release "Apo-Levocarb CR 100/25mg" at bedtime and an "Auro-Pramipexole 1.0 mg" with meals.
- Multi-centre, double-blinded parallel group, placebo-controlled study of creatine would soon come to a five-year close.
- Patient was on the placebo for the last five years.
- No conclusive results were evident in this research study.
- Dr. Suchowersky stated she would be leaving her position as Director and asked that a new neurologist, Dr. Tamara Pringsheim would take her place.

VR's Reaction and Insights

I was pleased that my condition has been somewhat stable over the last 7 years. I was also relieved that the research study ended with no conclusive results. Being on the placebo for five years was surprising and all for the better. I miss having Dr. Suchowersky as my neurologist. She was skilled and knowledgeable and very supportive of my efforts to combat PD.

April 30, 2014, I was assigned to a new neurologist, Dr. Tamara Pringsheim. Dr. Pringsheim is an assistant professor with the Department of Clinical Neurosciences, Psychiatry, Pediatrics and Community Health Sciences, at the University of Calgary's Faculty of Medicine. She is director of the Calgary Tourette and Pediatric Movement Disorder Clinic at the Alberta Children's Hospital. She provides care for patients at the Movement Disorder Clinic at the Foothills Medical Centre.

September 29, 2015, Dr. Pringsheim reported:
- The patient had no cognitive impairment.
- Experiences occasional constipation and urinary frequency.
- No pronounced postural (position) changes.
- There was no resting tremor or dyskinesias when examined in the office today.
- Barely detectable rigidity at the right elbow only.
- No evidence of bradykinesia in the upper or lower limbs.
- Gait revealed slight dystonic posturing of the right arm while walking.
- Altered medication slightly: "Apo-Levocarb 100/25mg" X 1 at 6 a.m., 10 a.m., 2 p.m., 6 p.m., 10 p.m. Take Mirapex 1 mg at 6 a.m., 2 p.m., 10 p.m.

March 10, 2015, Dr. Pringsheim communicated:
- No evidence of hypomimia (a reduced degree of facial expression) or hypophonia (soft speech) and extra ocular (eyes or vision movements were full with normal blink rate).
- Mild bradykinesia more evident in his arms and legs, with some mild cogwheel rigidly on the right more than the left.
- Able to rise out of a chair without using his arms.
- Coordination was normal to finger-to-nose bilaterally.
- Gait assessment showed no shuffling, freezing, or end bloc turns, and he had a normal base.

- Voluntarily moving his arms, more on the right than left.
- Doing well 8 years into his diagnosis of presumed idiopathic Parkinson's disease.
- Suggest a prescription for "Apo-Levocarb 100/25mg" five times daily (6:00 am, 9:00 am, 12 Noon, 4:00 pm, and 8:00 pm).
- Continue with Mirapex three times a day and warned him of potential side effects, including cognitive impairment, hallucinations, and impulse control disorder.

June 30, 2016, Dr. Pringsheim noted:
- No sign of resting tremor or any dyskinesias.
- Pain was evident in his right knee due to a meniscus tear.
- Mild rigidity on the right side only and mild bradykinesia bilaterally in all four limbs.
- Gait was normal except for some rigidity of the right arm while walking.
- Suggest a prescription of clonazepam or try over-the-counter melatonin for sleep.
- Adjust medication as needed.
- Prescribed Sinemet (100/25) mg one tablet 5x daily and Mirapex (1 mg 3x) daily.

VR's Reaction and Insights

To date, my new neurologist, Dr. Pringsheim is as skilled and knowledgeable as other doctors, but she has a completely different style. She is the kind of doctor who treats the whole patient and not just the symptoms. She is very thorough in her examinations and is a good listener and supportive of my condition. Often, she has a student doctor do the preliminary examination before providing her own assessment.

PART 5 - Nutrition

In Parts 5 and 6, I discuss the importance of a proper diet and exercise and the benefits that go beyond physical fitness and nutrition to bring relief from the stresses of living with a chronic, progressive disease.

I've found that a proper diet and certain nutrients enable my body to work more efficiently, have more energy, and help medications to work effectively.

Foods to Enjoy

According to Canada's Food Guide, about half of your food calories should come from the vegetable and fruit category. A healthy diet also includes a moderate portion of protein foods such as fish, and chicken, legumes and some dairy and moderate amounts of whole grains. Increase your water intake to between six and eight glasses daily and decrease your salt intake. Include bone strengthening nutrients such as calcium, magnesium, and vitamins D and K.

I try to eat properly. I've increased my water intake, which has its own problems during the night. I am basically a carnivore at heart. I love a good steak and baked potato but I continue to work at increasing my salad and vegetable intake. For me carbs are difficult to give up. Diet is always a work in progress. I do take a multivitamin daily as well as extra vitamin D3 and Lutein for my vision. Numerous studies have found significantly increased risks of Parkinson's in those that consume the highest amounts of dairy products compared to the lowest amounts, so I try to limit my consumption of milk and cheese.

There are many diets out there but not one that is geared specifically for those of us with Parkinson's. Some, such as the Mediterranean diet, have been linked with reduced risk of later onset and slower progression of PD in several studies. These foods are ones that have anti-inflammatory properties that help protect the brain from damage over time.

Foods to Avoid

Preservatives

There are over five thousand chemical additives that can be used in commercial food processing. Our bodies are simply not equipped to handle these artificial substances. Eliminating all of them is nearly impossible but you can be selective in what you consume.

Helpful Suggestions

I try to eat whole, unprocessed foods as much as possible. These are the foods my body was designed to handle. I try to purchase organically grown vegetables and fruits that haven't been treated with pesticides but that is almost impossible these days. I clean them well before I eat them.

Hormones in Meat

Most pork and chicken raised in Canada are without hormones. Beef is raised with hormones used to promote muscle growth and not fat growth.

Chemicalized and Processed Foods

As much as possible, buy organic fruits, vegetables, and grains to lower the amount of exposure you get to pesticides residues. Direct contact with herbicides and pesticides can put you at increased risk of PD.

Animal and Saturated Fats

Researchers have concluded that a high intake of animal fats is associated with a five-fold increase in risk of developing Parkinson's disease.

Salt

Excessive use of table salt (sodium chloride) effects the body in two different ways. It can deplete your body of potassium a mineral that's important to the proper functioning of the nervous system. It also can raise your blood pressure.

Helpful Suggestions

I have limited my intake of salt at the table. I always taste my food before salting it and try to use pepper for seasoning. Instead, I use sea salt, which is richer in minerals and less likely to drive up blood pressure. Remember that canned food is loaded with sodium chloride. It is better to choose fresh or frozen vegetables. Go light on the salt but never take it completely out of your diet because it is a necessary electrolyte.

Sugar

White sugar, brown sugar, and honey, break down very quickly into glucose. Our bodies are simply not equipped to process large amounts of sugar rapidly.

Spicy Foods

Foods seasoned with hot spices have been known to cause violent dyskinesia in some people of Parkinson's. As one who likes spicy food, I have reduced my intake.

Protein Restriction: Is It Necessary?

For some people, protein interferes with the effectiveness of their medication. The problem can be avoided by NOT eating high protein foods at the time medication is taken. It was recommended that I take my medication at least 30 minutes before meals although this is not always possible. Be sure to talk with your doctor about the timing of meals and meds to offset this problem.

Alcohol

Consult your doctor about drinking alcoholic beverages, as alcohol may interfere with some of your medications, or make you extra sleepy. For me, I have always enjoyed one glass of red wine with dinner. I haven't noticed any interference, but I do find myself napping during the occasional sports show on TV.

Additives and Sugar Substitutes

Parkinson's disease can be triggered or worsened by ingesting additives in some diet products, according to researchers.

Caffeine: Good or Bad?

Caffeine is a case in point. It has a stimulating effect on several different systems. It increases the level of the neurotransmitter norepinephrine in your brain causing you to feel alert and awake. However, too much caffeine in a chronically tense, aroused condition, leaves you more vulnerable to generalized anxiety. Caffeine is contained not only in coffee, but in many types of tea, cola beverages, chocolate, candy, cocoa, and over-the-counter drugs. Anxiety brings out the symptoms of PD. While I haven't eliminated caffeine altogether, I have reduced my consumption. I stick to decaffeinated tea after dinner.

Should I Add Supplements?

You may need to speak to your doctor about your specific needs. You may not need additional supplements other than what you get through a balanced diet. The nutritional treatment for Parkinson's disease is still a mystery.

Helpful Suggestions

As I mentioned above, I do take a multivitamin daily as well as extra vitamin D3 and Lutein for my vision. Many studies talk about adding vitamin supplements to your diet. Consult your doctor for his opinion.

Adding Vitamin B Complex may increase your dopamine levels. Vitamin E from foods such as nuts, wheat germ, spinach and other green vegetables may prove helpful.

Vitamin C is an antioxidant that helps in the production of dopamine. Magnesium is a mineral that acts as a natural relaxant. It may help relaxing muscles and enabling a PWP to get a better night sleep.

VR's Reaction and Insights

During my last examination with Dr. Pringsheim on March 21, 2017, I mentioned several changes that occurred in my life that raised my level of anxiety. Most significantly, my older brother passed away two weeks prior to my clinic visit. I also had total right knee replacement on May

24, 2017. No doubt, anxiety or low-level stress tends to increase the symptoms of PD.

March 21, 2017, Dr. Pringsheim gave an account:
- The patient is relatively stable with no significant changes since our last visit.
- No neck rigidity to the right upper extremity.
- Minimal bradykinesia in my right hand with finger tapping, hand movements, and pronation or postural supination.
- Able to arise from a chair without difficulty.
- Normal gait length and blog turning and arm swing.
- A slightly stooped posture.
- Pull-back test was negative.
- Discussion suggested that decreasing the total dose of pramipexole is necessary to prevent side effects as one gets older.
- Sinemet dose will remain the same.
- Pramipexole will decrease by a half-tablet at night and will continue with 1 mg in the morning and noon.

September 19, 2017, Dr. Pringsheim detailed:
- Good motor control throughout the day.
- Appeared to be in good health.
- Experiences occasional tremor in his right arm and leg at night after 10 p.m.
- No hallucinations or difficulties with cognition.
- No evidence of tremor during examination.
- No dyskinesia at rest.
- Tone was nearly normal bilaterally in the upper and lower limbs.
- Mild, barely detectable bradykinesia on the right side only.
- Gait examination was normal.

No progression of the disease since our last examination.

VR's Reaction and Insights

My manuscript lists many motor and non-motor symptoms in sections, Part 2-3. Reading information about the possible side effects is like reading a prescription warning. As I mentioned earlier, resting tremor, rigidity, and sleep disorder are major concerns. I have no difficulty falling asleep, but wake up every night somewhere around 3:00 to 4:00 A.M. My right side feels stiff and sometimes it is difficult to get back to sleep. Also, my right foot feels numb.

There is little doubt that taking medication causes one to dream. Vivid dreams yes, but no hallucinations, just silly dreams. Bladder and constipation are evident with PD. Frequency is a problem during the day, but not during sleep.

My mobility is good during the day but becomes more challenging during late evenings as I tire. Psoriasis (mainly scalp area) has been an annoyance for many years and sometimes is enhanced by Parkinson's disease. My dermatologist sees me on a regular basis every six months keeping my health issues in check. Dealing with Parkinson's disease definitely raises the level of anxiety and tends to elevate symptoms.

As I age, I find it important to supplement my diet with good vitamin add-ons, such as: a multi-vitamin for seniors, B12, Lutein for eye health, and D3.

PART 6 -
Power of Exercise

Part 6 demonstrates how the power of exercising does wonders for your health in general and in coping with Parkinson's disease.

Exercising regularly boosts the power of neurotransmitters in your brain to enhance your mood and ability to see life in a positive light. Exercise enhances your self-image by building confidence and dealing with life's stresses. People With Parkinson's (PWP) who exercise regularly seem to experience a milder and less-progressive disease process.

Exercise is vitally important for maintaining optimum motor function for all individuals and especially for individuals with Parkinson's disease. An exercise routine designed for the individual can compensate for the lack of movement caused by the disease. I try to plan my exercise routine and then change it up about one or two times a month so that I'm not bored. Stretching is particularly important since this is the best way to regularly achieve maximum range of movement in the joints and ligaments. I recommend you read "Parkinson's Disease & the Art of Moving" by John Argue. It includes excellent examples of exercises that you can do that are geared to PWP.

Helpful Suggestions

There are many types of exercises to choose from. For reducing generalized anxiety, aerobic exercise such as running, brisk walking, cycling outdoors, swimming, or aerobic dancing are most effective. To build muscle strength, you might want to include weightlifting weights, or isometric exercise such as wall plank or many of the yoga exercises. If socializing is important, then a team sport such as a racket sport, golf, baseball, volleyball, and skiing might serve your needs. If you like the outdoors, then hiking, or gardening would be appropriate. You can devote your efforts to working and trying to change the situation or devote your energy toward living the most fulfilling life you can. In my case, I try to do 30 to 60 minutes of endurance exercises (walking) every other day to maintain muscle control and tone helping to prevent rigidity.

VR's Reaction and Insights

One of the difficult motor symptoms that has caused me undue stress is rigidity or stiffness of muscles and joints. Stiffness is very noticeable either early morning or late at night. I work out at the local YMCA three to four times a week. I try to start at 7 A.M. for about one and one-half hours. I enjoy the social aspect working out with the same people currently. I mix the workout routines to stay motivated. To warm up, I use the stationary bike or treadmill for 20-30 minutes. I usually work out with partners who have their own medical issues, but I listen to music when working alone.

What happens when you are unable to work out at a fitness centre? I recommend working out at home or going for a walk or cycling outside. Inside, I have set up a stationary bike in-front of the television and tune the tv into a program that tours various cities. I enjoy the visual stimulation as well as the music playing in the background. I also use a workbench and dumbbells to complete my workout. I acquired these during COVID when I was unable to leave the house.

Walking provides the time and physical exercise to do my best thinking. I listen to music as a motivator to work out mental and emotional issues. One of my challenges is to walk different routes outside. I use music playlists to my advantage in motivating my walk.

While it isn't a physical exercise, challenging your mind is also very important. Activities such as teaching chess and card games to my grandchildren has been a very good stimulation. Attending a concert or mentoring a colleague that is diagnosed with a medical issue or chronic disease also can help to keep your brain cells active. Other mental activities might include recording your family history or enhancing your computer skills by organizing photo collections into albums. Accept that life with PD has no more certainty than life before PD. Choose to live in the present and not focus solely on the past or future.

PART 7 -
My Role in Clinical Trials

Part 7 discusses my role in three different research studies.

Should people diagnosed with Parkinson's disease become involved with clinical trials? If more people living with PD volunteer to participate in a trial, the testing and marketing periods (on average 12 to 15 years) can be reduced by a whopping 6 to 7 years. As such, new therapies can be available sooner and at lower cost. Very few - only 1% of PD patients - participate in a study as compared to 5% of the total cancer community.

The research team established certain qualifiers for selecting participants. For example, the study may include people over the age of 60 but exclude anyone under that age. Participants are selected and sign a document of informed consent placing them in a treatment group. The study may include one group for the experimental drug, one for an existing drug that's the current preferred treatment, and one for a placebo. Placebo is a medicine with no active ingredients; hence your symptoms remain unchanged. However, as many as 30% of the patients who receive a placebo in the trial report improvement. This result seems to be especially true in Parkinson's disease because just the possibility of getting a better medicine can create the expectation of a reward and liberate dopamine the chemical in your brain that controls movement.

Double blind studies are the preferred design for testing new therapies today because they ensure objectivity throughout the study. In double blind studies, participants don't know which treatment group, and the researcher doesn't know which group is getting the test therapy. In single-blind studies, only the participant or the researcher (but not both) knows which group is receiving the placebo and which is taking the actual drug. In open label studies, both the doctor and the study subject know what drug is administered.

Your signature on this document also indicates that you're aware of the risks, possible side effects, and potential benefits of the treatment. You have the right to withdraw from the trial any time you choose.

Research Studies

Research Study 1 - Investigational Drug SLV308 (March 20, 2007)

The title of the research study: A randomized double-blind, placebo-controlled-parallel group fixed and flexible SLV308[18] dose arm study to assess efficacy and safety of SLV308 monotherapy in the treatment of patients with early-stage Parkinson's disease. The principal investigator for this study was Dr. Oksana Suchowersky, Movement Disorders Program, University of Calgary.

VR's Reaction and Insights

In March of 2007, I took part in the above research study. It was an "investigational drug" since it was not an approved drug by Health Canada.

The first visit in March was a screening examination where I received a full medical examination measuring vital signs, weight, height, ECG, medical history and blood and urine sample. Beginning right away, I began taking the drugs. I didn't know whether I would receive the actual drug or a placebo. I took the two medication capsules three times a day. The dose increased over the first two weeks and further increased over the following two to five weeks. I was to contact the investigator if I wasn't feeling well. In addition to the trial drugs, I took my Parkinson's drugs, Mirapex and Sinemet. I was in drug overload. By early June

2007 I stopped taking the drugs because of negative side effects, sleep disturbance and lack of energy. Personally, I would not recommend any patient recently diagnosed with PD to join such a study in the first year of treatment. My understanding was that there were no conclusive results evident in this study.

Research Study 2 - Investigational Drug Creatine (November 2008)

The title of this study: A Multi-Centered, Double-Blinded, Parallel Group, Placebo Controlled Study of Creatine in Subjects with Treated Parkinson's disease.

This study evaluated whether the investigational drug creatine was able to slow the progression of Parkinson's disease. Creatine[19] had not been approved by the Food and Drug Administration to be used in treatment of PD. Two treatment groups were given either real or placebo packets of creatine powder. This investigational drug consisted of 10 grams of powder (one active and the other, placebo) for a period of 5 years.

VR's Reaction and Insights

I enjoyed being part of this research group as it didn't involve an experimental drug. Being part of a research group is a means of "paying forward" and contributing to help find a cure for PD. Also, I was examined much more frequently by the research team. Following the five-year study, I was surprised to learn that once again, there were no conclusive results. I also learned that I was in the placebo group. The one humorous thing about being in this study was that when I went through airport security when traveling I had to explain why I was bringing small, unmarked packets of white powder. It still provides a chuckle.

Research Study 3 - Ambulo-Sono (Music Walking Program) (September 4, 2013)

The title of this study: Music Walking Program for Parkinson's.

People with Parkinson's disease often show reduced leg and arm movement during walking. This is mainly because the size or amplitude of walking steps or arm swings tend to become smaller when not addressed. To prevent and treat gait disorders, a Calgary research team developed a Gait Reminder. This device used an iPod to calculate the step sizes during walking and used the size signals to trigger music play. When walking with larger steps the iPod played music. Steps that were shorter stopped the music play. In this way, the user was able to automatically maintain a consistent and normal step size during locomotion. The conditioning effect of music on the brain may also have helped create long term motor memory of automatic gait control. Music walking with large steps is a form of brisk exercise that can provide many additional health and medical benefits. The main purpose of the study was to develop a set of standard protocols or procedures.

VR's Reaction and Insights

I enjoyed being part of this research study as I listened to music while walking. This certainly was a motivational way of improving my overall gait. Unfortunately, I withdrew three years into the study because of knee pain issues. I still enjoy listening to my music when I am on the treadmill or walking track at the YMCA or at home. I choose upbeat music with a great rhythm.

PART 8 -
Introducing My Support Team

Part 8 introduces the importance of relying on a caring support team.

People with Parkinson's (PWP) must rely on both personal and professional help throughout the course of patient's illness. Each member of the support team has special talents and expertise that can help the patient manage symptoms and maintain normal function and quality of life.

My personal care team includes: my wife Jan; adult children Jeff and Jessica; daughter-in-law Melanie and son-in-law Gerrett are very supportive and helpful when needed. My grandchildren: Isaac, Zachery, and Caden provide me with much needed love and laughter. Others who may surprise with their willingness to help are relatives, close friends, and co-workers.

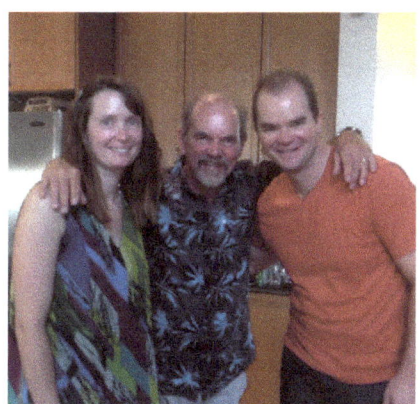 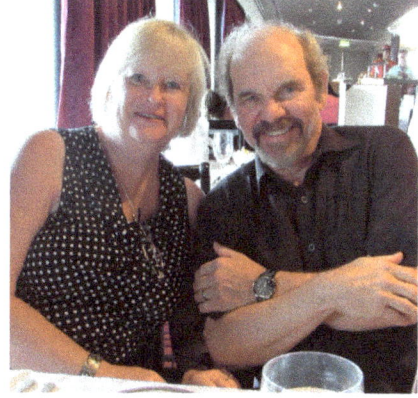

My professional care team includes: my primary care physician (PCP), neurologist, dermatologist, physiotherapist, massage therapist, and pharmacist. Each of these professionals have special talents and expertise that can help manage symptoms a maintain normal function and quality of life, often years following the initial diagnosis.

VR's Reaction and Insights

My wife, Jan plays a major role attending to my needs and acting as the main caretaker. She attends all medical appointments taking notes and asks questions.

I am truly grateful for the support received from each of my professionals. My primary care physicians (Dr. Kevin McCabe, Dr. Todd Leaman) have done an exceptional job in building a trust in support of my battle against PD. Both doctors were very knowledgeable, supportive, and took the time to answer all my questions. Presently, I have a new primary care physician, Dr. Raj.

Dr. Oksana Suchowersky has been my neurologist from 2007-2014. She was the Director of the Movement Disorder Clinic at the University of Calgary. She confirmed my PD condition on January 19, 2007. She encouraged me to become involved in three different clinical studies. Over seven years, we developed a positive rapport with each other. She was always attentive to my needs.

Dr. Tamara Pringsheim has been my neurologist since 2014. We've been together for almost 10 years. She is an Assistant Professor with the Department of Clinical Neurosciences at the University of Calgary. She has many qualities that I admire. She is knowledgeable, excellent communications skills, compassionate, inquisitive, and listens attentively.

Other specialists that play a more secondary role supporting my health include Dr. Stewart Adams (dermatologist), Dr. Rob Meloff (dentist), Wendy Kobelka (physiotherapist), Tammy Bock and Pamela Janz (massage therapists),

PART 9 -
Questions

Interests and Concerns

Being diagnosed with Parkinson's disease raises many questions that I would like to address and answer. These questions were derived from Ron Postuma's "Parkinson's Disease: An Introductory Guide," from Parkinson Canada and the Michael J. Fox Foundation documents, "Parkinson's 101 and Parkinson's 360[0.]"

Is Parkinson's Research important?

For me, taking part in clinical studies was a chance to "pay it forward" for others who will follow. I felt that it was my way of contributing to the discovery of a cure for PD. My own personal PD research gave me a better understanding of the disease itself and a more effective means to share with my family, friends, and others diagnosed with this chronic disease.

Is the Parkinson's Disease Rating Scale (UPDRS) a true predictor that a person has PD?

In 2007, I was examined by two medical apprentices using the (UPDRS[20]) method to determine whether I had PD. This widely used motor component of UPDRS, which takes about 30 minutes, covers fourteen categories where muscles may be behaving badly, including speech, facial expression, tremor, rigidity, finger tapping, ability to rise from a chair, posture, gait, and balance. The aggregate score (between 0 and 108) is supposed to quantify a patients' motor condition and reach a conclusion that he/she has PD.

What do the critics say about the Rating Scale? Is it accurate?

While some neurologists and researchers defend it, others privately mock it as a poor representation snapshot of the patient's physical state. Neurologists see their patients every six months for a thirty-minute session and thus spend every year a total of one hour being observed. That leaves "8,765 hours" when PD is not being monitored. The test is highly subjective as well. Quite frankly, I was in denial for well over a year because of this simplistic method to determine if I had PD. I did and I do.

What PD medication is right for you?

Parkinson's medications work in different ways. Many are pills that you swallow, but some can be given through skin patches or intestinal infusions. Over time, as symptoms progressed or complications arose, my neurologist adjusted my medications. The dosage was changed as well as the timing of when I took my pills. I have been on Sinemet since the beginning. This is the "gold standard" of Parkinson's medication. I try to stay in tune with my symptoms and keep track of which ones are most bothersome. I also keep track of which medications I am taking and how well medication is or is not working. This information has been very helpful for my neurologist when I have my semi-annual meeting.

Can I take generic pills or is it best to take name-brand medications?

A generic medicine is required to be the same as a brand-name medicine in dosage, safety, effectiveness, strength, stability, and quality, as well as in the way it is taken. Over the years, I have found little or no difference between brands. I am currently taking a generic version of Sinemet.

What should I do if I'm late taking my medication?

Do not take a double dose to make up for the dose that you missed. If it is almost time for the next dose, skip the missed dose and take the next one when it is due. Best thing is to take your dose as soon as you remember. You will need to adjust the schedule for the pills you need to take over the rest of the day.

Otherwise, take it as soon as it is remembered, and then go back to taking the medicine as usual. I have a timer that reminds me when to take my pills at a set interval. It is only as accurate as the person using and that's me.

Is Parkinson's genetic or hereditary?

We do not know exactly what causes Parkinson's nation of genetic and environmental factors are the cause. Genetics causes about 10% to 15% of all PWP. Understanding the connection between Parkinson's and genetics can help us understand how the disease develops. There is no one else in my family, past or present with PD that I know of.

What kinds of pain can be part of PD?

Parkinson's patients suffer from the same pain other people have, which is often amplified by Parkinson's motor dysfunction, but they can also have additional pain problems unique to PD. Lower back pain and back of the neck pain are most common. I went initially to my doctor with a tremor in my right foot and a very sore right shoulder. From there my journey began. I find that strengthening exercises and stretching are helpful.

Should I try medical marijuana as a means of reducing the symptoms of PD?

I raised this topic with my neurologist. Do I have particular symptoms that may be amenable to treatment with medical marijuana? She wasn't against my taking it but would want to carefully monitor my reaction to it. She felt that it was expensive and not always effective and perhaps not needed at this time.

Although the medications that doctors prescribe can be helpful, there remain gaps in what the medications can treat. Understandably, people with PD are eager to find alternative methods to help manage their symptoms, leading many of these patients to look into whether other therapies, such as medical marijuana, also known as medical cannabis, can be useful.

Does Levodopa and Protein cause medication absorption concerns?

Levodopa continues to be the gold standard for treatment of Parkinson's disease (PD), and nearly everyone diagnosed with PD is prescribed this medication. I haven't really investigated this concern. I tend to take my medications on a timer regulated schedule. I have cut down on my red meat consumption. Not everyone with PD has this problem.

Is it okay for me to drive if I have PD?

What I have come to realize over the years is that PD is a very individualized disease. It differs from person to person. Because driving is a complex activity that requires my full attention, physically, mentally and emotionally, PD can affect my driving. Fortunately, my back-up driver is willing to take me wherever I want to go. If I feel there is a concern, I let her drive. Your neurologist is responsible for identifying and assessing drivers who may be unfit to drive.

How are "On-Off "Fluctuations treated?

My usual signs of wearing off are slowness of movement or an increase in tremor before my next dose of medication is due. But wearing off can also increase other symptoms associated with Parkinson's, including fatigue and pain from dystonia (muscle contractions). I have experienced all of this.

The goal of managing motor fluctuations and dyskinesias is to help you remain as active and independent as possible. Your neurologist may adjust the dosage of levodopa either by adjusting the dosage or its frequency. She may add different medications to your current regime to help keep the levels of dopamine more consistent to avoid "off-time". My neurologist has adjusted the frequency several times over the years. In doing that she has also adjusted the total daily dosage.

Why do motor fluctuations happen?

As PD progresses, it is common for more dopamine producing brain cells to die, causing the benefits from Parkinson's medication to not last as long as they did before. Eventually you reach a point where your brain stops producing dopamine in large amounts and therefore must rely on the medicine to compensate. Researchers think this happens for two reasons: One is cells become less able to store dopamine. When this occurs, the cells fade. Two the cells are unable to release dopamine without medications, such as levodopa. When the dosage wears off, about three to four hours after taking it, there is no more, resulting in worsening of your symptoms.

Can I travel with Parkinson's?

I love to travel and had numerous trips despite Parkinson's. In fact, the PD symptoms were less obvious during the trips. You can travel without restrictions as long as you do not have advanced PD. Make sure you have travel insurance, and that you share all medical information with the insurance company.

Is it possible to find a cure for PD? Are there new treatments to slow the progression?

While there are many active areas of research with lots of promise, currently, there is no cure for Parkinson's disease. There are many resources and options available, and there's a growing field of research into the disease. Every day, researchers are studying new therapies and potential cures. I did my part in the three studies in which I participated.

What are the early signs of Parkinson's Disease?

No single one of these signs means that you should worry, but if you have more than one, consider speaking with your doctor. In my case, I noticed my right foot shaking when tired near the end of the day. About four months later, I felt a soreness in my right shoulder. Early signs include tremor in your hand, finger, foot or toes; change in handwriting showing smaller letter sizes; loss of smell in foods such as bananas, dill pickles or liquorice; trouble sleeping and acting out dreams when you are deeply asleep; stiffness in your joints.

Is Your Blood Pressure affected by Parkinson's?

Some people with PD may have problems with low blood pressure, called hypotension. Orthostatic hypotension is a sharp drop in blood pressure that happens when a person gets up from bed or a chair, causing dizziness or even loss of consciousness. People with PD who have a combination of orthostatic hypotension and impairment of postural reflexes (loss of balance) are at risk for dizziness, fainting, and falls leading to fractures. Lying down and standing blood pressure recordings are essential as diagnostic measures. I've only experienced one episode of fainting due to low blood pressure.

Is vertigo a sign or symptom of Parkinson's Disease?

Vertigo and dizziness are commonly reported symptoms in people with Parkinson's. Most experts agree that dizziness and vertigo can be broadly defined as the sensation of spinning or whirling, and the sensation can be associated with balance problems. I failed to notice this phenomenon until many years after being diagnosed.

What should I expect from treatment with dopamine medications?

In general, it depends on the type of treatment you have. When I first started taking Sinemet I noticed an almost immediate improvement in my movement and muscle control (e.g., less stiffness, faster walking, clearer voice, and more). Sinemet helped to improve my tremor. I started to feel myself again.

Can Parkinson's impact you emotionally causing anxiety?

PD is known to influence many aspects of the movement; studies have shown the two non-motor symptoms anxiety and depression play a key role in the disease and have the greatest impact on overall health. Like most people, I tend to worry about things I have no control over. Fortunately, there are proven strategies, including mindfulness, meditation and exercises that can help manage my anxiety.

VR's Reaction and Insights

I have not experienced "dose failures," defined as when your medication doesn't work at all. To date, I have had no serious issues. I do forget to take medication when involved with numerous tasks. I've purchased a timing reminder to keep me on track. It is very loud.

I do worry about losing my license to drive. However, I am very cognizant about driving if the symptoms are noticeable. I do not hesitate in asking someone else to take the wheel. Recently, I underwent a medical examination and eye test to determine being fit to drive at seventy-five years of age. My driver's license has been extended for five years.

I do and do not take my medication at prescribed times during the day. I use an electronic device to monitor taking meds at three and one-half hours apart. This does not always begin with breakfast, lunch or dinner times. Taking meds at a specific time depends on when I start my day and workout times.

My neurologist suggested I could give marijuana oil a try, but only if she monitors this approach. It is costly and comes in the form of a liquid oil. I need to have further discussion with my neurologist on this topic.

I am very much in favour of being part of research studies that might find a cure for the disease or slow the progression. I've been involved with three different studies that you can read about in the appendix. I like the idea of sharing with others knowledge of the disease and how it affects me personally.

March 6, 2018, Dr. Pringsheim communicated:
- The patient was alert and appropriate throughout the examination.
- On cranial nerve examination, pupils were equal and reactive to light.
- No RAPD
- Fundoscopy (examining the inside of the eye) was normal. Visual acuity and fields were normal. Extra-ocular movements were full.
- Facial sensation and muscle movements were symmetric. Palate and tongue were midline.

- Hearing was grossly normal. Sternocleidomastoid (muscles that control the neck) and trap strength were full. Tongue strength was full.
- On motor examination, he had normal bulk, tone, and strength.
- He did have a mild resting tremor in his right hand with distraction.
- Mild bradykinesia in his upper and lower extremity. Reflexes were 2+ throughout with downing toes. Sensation was grossly normal to temperature and touch.
- Finger to nose was grossly (extremely) normal with some mild tremor his right hand. On gait examination, he had a slight abnormal movement of his right arm but was otherwise normal.
- On Romberg he had mild drift backwards.
- No significant changes currently, however, continue our slow wean off the pramipexole.
- Continue Sinemet 100/25 mg 6 times per day. Decrease pramipexole to 1 mg b.i.d.
- He was told to contact us should he have any questions and concerns about his condition.

VR's Reaction and Insights

What am I experiencing as of October 2018? Rigidity and tremor are more noticeable on my right side. Tremor becomes more evident when feeling anxious. Normally, go to bed around 10:30 PM and easily fall asleep. Wake up numerous times during the night. Sometimes I take one Sinemet tablet around 4 or 5 A.M. to alleviate stiffness. No issues with dyskinesias. Silly dreams are always part of my night's sleep. No feelings of depression but feel anxious more than usual. I should consider myself fortunate that progression has been slow after twelve years.

I continue to maintain a regular schedule dealing with tasks around the house. I work out at the Crowfoot YMCA 4-5 times per week. I play golf during the summer and look forward to skiing in winter. I also play guitar and travel throughout the year. I spend a great deal of time on the computer keeping my cognitive skills in tack.

October 11, 2018, Dr. Pringsheim reported:

- The patient appears well with a resting tremor affecting his jaw and right side (high amplitude and low frequency tremor).
- Memory is good and does not experience hallucinations.
- Mild rigidity on right side as well as bradykinesia.
- Examined feet and did not find any convincing sensory defects in either lower limb.
- Continue to withdraw Mirapex to 0.5 mg three times daily.
- Increasing levodopa to 1 1/2 mg five times daily.
- Medication prescribed Sinemet (100/25) mg one tablet five times daily and Mirapex 1 mg and 0.5 mg in the afternoon and evening.
- Encouraged Vic to try reading/practicing mindfulness for his anxiety.
- Reassured Vic that he is doing well.

VR's Reaction and Insights

What am I experiencing since my last examination on October 11, 2018? I have noted minor progression of the disease. Both resting tremor and rigidity remain main concerns. Resting tremor is more noticeable when feeling anxious. When travelling and on vacation, the symptoms appear less of a problem. Rigidity is more evident in my trunk (lower back and buttocks) area, especially in early morning. On occasion, my right knee feels stiff and right foot feels numb. Sometimes medication takes 15-20 minutes to take effect and lasts for about 3 1/2 hours. I am not experiencing any dyskinesias or difficulty with my gait. General mood is good and described as upbeat. I have not experienced any falls to date and no memory or cognitive issues. I find it difficult to fall into a deep sleep, but the clonazepam does help suppress vivid dreams. I continue to remain active exercising 4-5 times per week. To sharpen my cognitive skills, I attempt to play guitar, electric keyboard and golf. I've also decided to increase my walking outdoors on a regular schedule.

April 30, 2019, Dr. Pringsheim outlined:

- On physical examination, the patient appeared well.

- There was a resting tremor affecting the right upper limb.
- No dyskinesias at rest or provoked through examination.
- Very mild rigidity bilaterally.
- Minimal bradykinesia of all four limbs.
- Gait was normal.
- Suggested getting mild anxiety under control as it seems to have an impact on his motor symptoms.
- Recommended that he try mindfulness-based cognitive theory for his anxiety.
- Might try cannabidiol oil as another solution.
- Currently taking Sinemet (100/25) mg 1 1/2 tablets five times daily, Mirapex 0.5 mg three times daily, and clonazepam 0.5 mg at bedtime.

VR's Reaction and Insights

My next visit and examination with Dr. Pringsheim was scheduled for October 29, 2019. Unfortunately, I received a letter during the summer that Dr. Tamara Pringsheim had taken a leave of absence because of illness. It was hoped that she would return to the clinic when her condition improves.

Another neurologist, Dr. Sarah Furtado had graciously accepted to be her replacement until she returned. I was scheduled to meet with Dr Furtado on Tuesday, October 29, 2019, at 9:00 A.M. in Health Science Centre, 1st Floor Area 3.

October 29, 2019, Dr. Sarah Furtado substituting for Dr. Pringsheim, summarized the patient's condition:
- The patient has a remarkable history dating back to January 19, 2007.
- He continues with Sinemet regular (100/25), 1 1/2 tablets each at 5:00, 9:00, AM 12:00 Noon, 4:00, and 8:00 PM.
- Also, Mirapex 0.25 mg two tablets each at 9:00 AM, 12:00 PM and 4:00 PM.

- At bedtime, he may choose to take 0.5 clonazepam or administer 5 gm of Melatonin to help him with a regular sleep pattern.
- He admits suggested times become disjointed when busy working on different projects.
- Medications kick in within 15-20 minutes and sometimes wear off before the next scheduled dosage.
- He does not have dyskinesias, but experiences resting tremor during wear off times.
- He has no postural hypotension, no hallucinations, and no confusion.
- Rested sleep continues to be bothersome waking up around 3:00 A.M.
- On examination, I noticed a slight diminishment in facial expression and voice volume.
- No resting tremor, but mild bradykinesia.
- No dyskinesias, good stride length and arm swing.
- During this hour and one-half examination, I reinforced that he is doing quite well.
- I emphasized him to try taking medications on a more regular basis.
- I renewed his medications and will see him in six months' time.

VR's Reaction and Insights

As of January 19, 2020, I will have dealt with Parkinson's disease for 13 years. I must admit to being anxious having to be examined by a new neurologist substituting for Dr. Pringsheim.

The question remains: "What motor and non-motor symptoms continue to appear troublesome up to January 19, 2020?" Rigidity and resting tremor are the main culprits. Rigidity is more evident in the trunk region (lower back and buttocks) area. Resting tremor is more evident when tired or getting out of bed in the early morning. Normal sleep patterns are disrupted because of lack of medication while sleeping. Dr. Furtado suggested chewing on one tablet of Sinemet may help me return to a more normal sleep pattern. I should also mention that my meeting and examination with Dr. Furtado was extremely positive as she showed a caring and professional interest in my condition.

I would imagine feeling fortunate that many of the other PD symptoms are either mild or non-existent. Cognitive skills remained focused. I am not experiencing any dyskinesias or difficulty with my gait. Overall, my general mood is good and described as up-beat. I admit that a noticeable progression of overall symptoms sometimes caused anxiety. I am also aware that my central nervous system is much more sensitive as the result of PD disease. Anxiety can intensify my over-all condition. I continue to remain active exercising 4-5 times per week at the local YMCA. To sharpen my cognitive skills, I attempted to play guitar and piano. During the summer, I tried to play golf on a more regular basis.

Recently, I was concerned that my left knee was causing me issues. The right knee was replaced in 2017. I would like to increase the range of motion, flexibility, strength, endurance, and balance to both knees. The most important factor in dealing PD symptoms is through exercise. As such, I have taken the initiative to be re-examined by Sports Medicine, Dr. Jim Thorne, Group23 located in Canada Olympic Park in Calgary. After a thorough examination last week, Dr. Thorne stated I was in good physical shape and the left knee was not serious. Dr. Thorne, along with physiotherapist, Wendy Kobelka will develop a plan to improve both knees and overall conditioning.

November 26, 2020, Dr. Tamara Pringsheim summarized the patient's condition using the platform Zoom as a result of the Covid-19 virus:

- Currently taking levodopa two tablets at 9:00 A.M., 12:00 Noon, 4:00 P.M., 8:00 P.M. and one tablet at 5:00 A.M.
- He also takes 0.5 pramipexole tablet at 9:00 A.M. and 4:00 P.M., and 0.25 mg at 1:00 P.M.
- Also, takes 0.5 mg clonazepam at bedtime.
- Decreased pramipexole dosage at 1:00 P.M. from 0.5 to 0.25 mg. There has been no detrimental effect decreasing this dosage.
- Increased levodopa slightly by half-tablet at each dose except for the 5:00 A.M. dosage.
- He reported his motor functions overall were good. He does experience tremor, bradykinesia, and rigidity, especially when

his medication levels start to level off. Tremor will increase when anxiety increases.
- Does not experience hallucinations or delusions.
- No history of REM sleep behaviour disorder.
- Sometimes feels light-headed after taking his levodopa.
- Reported an increase in anxiety in the setting of the pandemic.
- Blood pressure appeared normal range. At the beginning of my visit there was a resting tremor affecting his jaw and right arm. Over the course of his visit, these started to diminish.
- Will decrease his pramipexole by omitting the 1:00 P.M. dosage.
- Suggested mindfulness-based stress reduction for the treatment of anxiety,

July 6, 2021, Dr. Tamara Pringsheim summarized the patient condition at the Movement Disorder Clinic at Foothills Medical Centre:
- Currently taking levodopa two tablets at 9:00 A.M., 12:00 Noon, 4:00 P.M., 8:00 P.M. and one tablet at 5:00 A.M.
- He also takes pramipexole 0.5 mg at 9:00 A.M. and 4:00 P.M., and 0.5 mg clonazepam at bedtime.
- Overall, he is doing quite well.
- Anxiety tends to exacerbate his symptoms of PD.
- He is now double vaccinated against COVID and feels more confident in dealing with the Covid -19.
- In our last visit, I decreased his pramipexole by 0.25 mg.
- He reports no motor impact from this reduction.
- Reports some worsening of resting tremor in context of feeling anxious and stressed.
- He has not experienced any falls.
- Does have a resting tremor, mainly on his right side as well as affecting his jaw.
- He states never experiencing dyskinesias.
- Experiences vivid dreams but does not move about the bed or call out at night.
- Bowel movement is good daily. Some urinary frequency throughout the day, but only once during nighttime. Some issues with syncope or pre syncope.

- On physical examination, he appeared quite well. There was some tremor in his jaw and right arm and leg.
- Examined him five minutes after he took his levodopa resulting in mild rigidity bilaterally, which was most prominent on his right side, as well as mild bradykinesia with repetitive movements of the upper lower limbs.
- Gait examination was essentially normal.
- He is a 76-year-old man with a 15-year history of Parkinson's disease.
- Overall, I think the patient is doing quite well.
- No recommended changes to his medication currently.

October 25, 2022

- Signs indicate that he is doing well. He can maintain all tasks around the house. He keeps himself active by exercising on a regular basis at the YMCA. He plays golf in the spring and summer.
- I asked the patient what symptoms he was experiencing since our last meeting.
- He stated that he was somewhat anxious due to the Global Pandemic, his brother's death, and being told by his family doctor that he was leaving the profession.
- He mentioned that he was writing a book about his journey with PD. He felt the added burden of researching and writing about PD increased his anxiety.
- I reinforced that anxiety is quite normal. Especially, if a person is diagnosed with a chronic disease.
- I tested his coordination and balance while observing his walk, stance, sit, turn, extend my arms and hands, and so on.
- Vic is not experiencing and hallucinations or paranoid thinking. He reports that his mood is good. He has not fainted.
- Occasionally, he feels light-headed. He does not suffer from constipation. He has mild urinary urgency during the day and to get up once or twice to go to the bathroom.
- He notes that his writing is becoming a bit micrographic.
- By the end of the day, he noticed that his voice decreases slightly.

- On physical examination, Vic appeared in good health. I did not notice any tremor or dyskinesias at rest.
- There was barely detectable rigidity in the arms and barely detectable bradykinesia with receptive movements of the arms and legs. Gait examination was nearly normal.
- Overall, I feel Vic is doing extremely well with resect of PD.
- I think one of his biggest struggles is anxiety related to his health condition.
- I have done my very best to try to reassure Vic is taking excellent care of himself.

VR's Reaction and Insights

Symptoms are what you tell your neurologist as opposed to signs what your neurologist observes during the examination. I was pleased that her observations were positive. Again, she emphasized that I was doing well, and few could tell I had Parkinson's disease. I talked about loss of weight (5 pounds). She said that it is normal as one ages. I mentioned that I was examined by a doctor at Group 23 at Canada Olympic Park to check my knee replacement. He would see me again in April 2023. I've tried to increase my range of motion so that I can ski and make use of my bicycle.

The last two and one-half years have been stressful because of the Global Pandemic and Covid-19. My brother passed away at the start of Covid-19. Sad to say that my family doctor has decided to leave the profession. Finding a new doctor has been a stressful task.I asked my neurologist whether the drug called clonazepam 0.5 mg taken every night is addictive.

May 16, 2023
- Vic is taking levodopa two tablets at 9:00 a.m., 12:00 p.m., 4:00 p.m., and 8:00 p.m., and one tablet at 10:30 p.m. and 4:00 a.m. He is also taking pramipexole 0.375 mg twice daily and clonazepam 0.5 mg at bedtime.
- He feels his tremor and stiffness have increased on his right side.

- He states that his main symptom of his levodopa wearing off is the emergence of a right-sided tremor affecting his arm and leg, as well as stiffness.
- He states that the duration of the levodopa response tends to vary depending on his activity level.
- He feels that his symptoms are worse when he is anxious about something.
- Sometimes he forgets to take his medications when he is busy. Uses a dose set box to keep track of them.
- Wearing off time is much the same as before about 3 1/2 hours.
- Increased anxiety due to continuing to write his book about Parkinson's. He stated that it is nearly finished.
- Managing his anxiety by taking breaks and doing something else certainly helps.
- He feels that his typing skills have got worse and creates a feeling of anxiety. Also, deals with continually revising his work.
- No difficulties with memory, no hallucinations, or delusions, or with impulse control
- Not shuffling his feet except in early morning. Body is stiff when he gets up. Is careful about going down the stairs.
- Tense in the right arm but other tests are fine.
- On physical examination, Vic appeared well. Blood pressure was 140/86. His heart rate in sitting position was 95.
- Throughout our encounter, Vic experienced a jaw tremor and a right leg tremor. There was mild bradykinesia on right side. Gait examination was normal.
- Overall, I feel Vic is doing quite well. I do not see any need to change his dosages.
- Eventually, we will discontinue the pramipexole completely.
- He is not having sighs of cognitive dysfunction, hallucinations, or impulse control disorders, so I do not feel the need to further lower his dosage of pramipexole at this visit.
- I have encouraged Vic to remain active. I plan to see him in the follow-up in 6 months.

- We talked about new treatment coming out next year - a subcutaneous leva-dopa injection.

VR's Reaction and Insights

There is no change in my medications. I'm pleased. When Dr. Leaman left I was able to find a doctor by the name of Dr. S. Raj. My neurologist knows of her and states that she has a good reputation. I've been feeling more anxiety of late probably due to writing this manuscript. I've learned a lot about Parkinson's in doing my research. I sincerely hope that others will benefit reading this manuscript and choosing their own right road in helping others.

Epilogue

"The Road Not Taken" is one of my favourite poems, by American poet, Robert Frost. Which path should I choose? A path that includes fear of the unknown, disbelief, gloom, and unhappiness after being diagnosed with Parkinson's disease. Or a path that reflects hope, a positive attitude, a challenge in life and a change of lifestyle? I choose the latter, supported by the people that care. My immediate family that includes an exceptional wife, two amazing adult children, a supportive daughter in-law, son in-law, and three loving grandsons. A support team that also includes friends and medical practitioners.

Some Final Thoughts:

Attitude can very well be the difference between taking control of this disease and allowing PD to control you.

You have the right prescription to make an enormous difference in your emotional state of mind and self-image.

Exercise daily. Do something, walk somewhere, join a gym and then go.

Eat and drink wisely. Lessen stimulants (such as caffeine and chocolate) that can contribute your anxiety.

Find joy in everything you do. Laugh daily. It increases dopamine production.

Surround yourself with people who are positive, optimistic, and upbeat.

Accept and work through circumstances and challenges that you can control.

Practice mindfulness. Live in the present. You can't change the past and you don't know what the future will bring.

Pay it Forward. Participate in research that advances the study of Parkinson's.

Look again at the cover of this book and ask yourself whether you have the strength and courage to accept your fate and make changes to your lifestyle. Live in the present ...

Appendices

APPENDIX 1: Timeline

Timeline

This timeline is an accurate comparison of observations made by my neurologist following each medical examination. It provides me the opportunity to draw conclusions based on my own reaction and insights throughout my Parkinson's journey.

January 19, 2007, to March 27, 2023

January 19, 2007, Dr. Suchowersky's Neurologist Report
- The patient's diagnosed with Parkinson's Disease.
- Prescribed a dopamine agonist, amantadine widely used to treat mild cases of Parkinson's.
- This drug has been known to speed up recovery of flu like conditions as the result of a viral infection.

VR's Reaction and Insights

As a result, I experienced negative responses. I had difficulty sleeping waking up every two hours. The right side of my body felt stiff and uncomfortable. I experienced disturbing dreams. I was prescribed amantadine, trazodone for sleep, and an unknown experimental drug as part of the research.

On the advice of Dr. Suchowersky, I would enter a Titration research study. April 2007, I felt nauseous, stiffness in shoulders, and loss of energy.

Mid-June 2007 On-Call Neurologist.
- An on-call neurologist prescribed omeprazole for the patient's chest and domperidone for stomach cramps.

VR's Reaction and Insights

My symptoms got worse as I felt a heaviness in my chest, dizziness, stiffness in both hand, and severe headaches. I asked to be withdrawn from the Titration research study.

June 15, 2007, Dr. Suchowersky
- The Titration study closed due to several issues.
- The patient's negative reaction may be the result given the highest dosage.
- No conclusive findings were evident from the study.
- Prescribed Levo-Carb or Sinemet (100 x 25 mg) 1 tab three times daily at meals.
- As part of the follow up program, he would see the resident Psychiatrist, Dr. Quickfall.

June 22, 2007, Dr. Jeremy Quickfall Psychiatrist Sport
- The patient's anxiety mostly limited to his illness.
- Thought form was linear and goal directed.
- No abnormal content.
- He showed himself to be very intelligent and articulate man.
- Lot of insights into his own condition/and motivation to address them.
- No obvious perceptual or cognitive impairments.
- Recommend positive coping mechanisms using yoga and meditation.
- Deal with anxiety with non-pharmacological means as much as possible.

- Suggested reading the "Anxiety & Phobia Workbook" to control symptoms.
- Prescribed low strength 0.5 mg anti-van for anxiety to be taken when needed.
- Suggest a follow-up visit in two months.

August 22, 2007
- The patient's anxiety has remarkably improved.
- Taking trazodone nightly helped his sleep cycle.
- Overall anxiety is a combination of adjustment to his illness, adverse effects of medications, and detailed-oriented coping style.
- No underlying acute anxiety disorder requiring separate treatment is needed.
- No follow-up is required currently.

VR's Reaction and Insights

I was pleased with Dr. Quickfall's assessment and recommendations as my condition improved immensely over summer months. The medication prescribed earlier by Dr. Suchowersky appeared to be working. My acceptance and willingness to adapt to a new lifestyle was about to begin.

August 23, 2007
- These are some of the questions I asked but received no definitive answers. I asked, "Why me?" Again, limited response as there was no history of PD in my family.
- "What causes Parkinson's disease?" One theory suggests some toxin in the environment triggered a gene that resulted in the loss of "dopamine" in an area of the brain.
- "Is it hereditary?" Again, a limited response suggesting that it is probably more the environment.
- "Is there any margin of error in the neurologist's diagnosis?" I must admit that looking at the various stages of progression enhances one's fear of the consequences.
- I was surprised that my neurologist performed simple physical tests in diagnosing the disease.

- "Did the diagnosis raise my level of anxiety?" It's not a death sentence, but definitely there is a need to make significant changes in one's lifestyle.
- "Was I in denial?" You bet, and it lasted for over a year. I've always set goals for myself in a positive manner dealing with life's challenges. I couldn't accept defeat, so I focused on learning more about the disease.

May 19, 2010, Dr. Suchowersky
- The patient is experiencing mild Parkinson's disease symptoms which is reasonably controlled with medication.
- He has agreed to take part in a Double-Blinded Placebo control trial using Creatinine in hopes to slow down progression of PD (appendix 2).
- Continue taking Sinemet (100/25) mg x3 with meals and Sinemet CR (100/25) mg x 1 a slow-release tablet at bedtime.

VR's Reaction and Insights

I agreed with Dr. Suchowersky's suggestions and look forward to this second research study as it doesn't involve taking drugs. I like to believe that taking part in research may help others that are dealing with Parkinson's.

Since the beginning of my diagnosis, both resting tremor and rigidity are most notable symptoms. Being tired or stressed makes matters worse. Since its discovery, Levo-Carb is known as the "gold standard" treatment for this disease. And yes, a glass of wine or two, does help relax the body and calm these symptoms. Rigidity is also quite evident especially in the right hand and trunk area of the body. To date, I have not experienced bradykinesia or issues involving balance.

To keep this condition under control, I work out at the Crowfoot YMCA 4-5 times per week. Exercise on a regular basis is paramount in dealing with PD.

Extension of Part 3 Non-Motor Symptoms

VR's Reaction and Insights

What non-motor symptoms have I had to deal with since early diagnosis? Anxiety is the main culprit. It appears to be intensified because it affects the central nervous system.

I also admit being in denial during the first two years of the disease. I sometimes worry about blood pressure being too low. After workouts, my resting pulse is constant at 60 beats per minute. However, the 60 beats per minute may be an indication of being physically fit.

Being tired watching television late at night can cause double vision. This has been corrected by removing cataracts and inserting new lenses. My vision is now 20/20 and I use low strength reading glasses for close work. Was this caused by Parkinson's or is it simply the aging process?

I've noticed that my writing has been affected because of PD. Constipation is also an occasional concern. I've dealt with minor scalp psoriasis over the years and see a dermatologist every six months. Sex problems tend to occur because of age, but PD can make it even more difficult. For men, drugs such as Viagra can make a significant difference to enjoy intimate relationships.

Since the beginning of my battle with Parkinson's, sleep has been a real issue. I usually go to bed about 10 P.M. and have little difficulty falling asleep. Unfortunately, I wake up around 2:30 to 3:30 A.M. At this point, the medication has worn off, so I sense tremor and rigidity. I either read for one hour or listen to music. Sometimes I fall back to sleep, and other times am forced to take one capsule of levo-carb. I've tried mild medication prescribed by the neurologist or over the counter sleep medication such as melatonin. Sleep continues to be a concern.

After reviewing both motor and non-motor symptoms, I have concluded that symptoms are difficult to compare as no two individuals are alike with Parkinson's.

October 26, 2011, Dr. Suchowersky
- The patient is doing well with respect to PD. There is minimal progression of symptoms over last four years.

- He should continue to take Sinemet 100/25 mg along with breakfast, lunch and dinner, Sinemet CR 200 mg at bedtime and Mirapex 0.75 mg with meals.

VR's Reaction and Insights

I noticed a slight increase in resting tremor when trying to sleep. I also reported rigidity or tightness of muscles in my right hand/arm and lower back. Again, sleep disturbance has been an issue since being diagnosed. I have no trouble falling asleep but wake up about 3 o'clock feeling a tremor and stiffness in my trunk area.

November 7, 2012, Dr. Suchowersky
- No side effects taking creatine for the last five years as part of a research study.
- Condition is stable with respect to PD.
- No gait or balance issues.
- Continue to take Sinemet 100/25 mg and Sinemet CR 200/25 at bedtime along with Mirapex 0.75 mg at breakfast, lunch and dinner.

VR's Reaction and Insights

I've noticed an increase in tremor on my right side. This occurs mostly in morning or late evening when feeling tired. No evidence of bradykinesia, impaired balance, or cognitive issues. A restful sleep remains my main concern.

October 11, 2013, Dr. Suchowersky
- Progression was minimal over the last six years.
- Medication shows very little change taking Sinemet 100/25 mg with meals, Mirapex 1 mg with meals, and Sinemet CR 200 at bedtime.
- Multi-centre, double-blinded parallel group, placebo-controlled study of creatine would soon come to a five-year close.
- Nothing conclusive was evident in the findings.

- He was on the placebo for the last 5 years.
- Dr. Suchowersky is leaving her position as Director and asked that Dr. Tamara Pringsheim would take her place.

VR's Reaction and Insights

I am pleased that my condition has been somewhat stable over the last six years. I was also thankful that the research study has ended with no conclusive results. Being on the placebo for five years was surprising and all for the better. I look forward meeting Dr. Pringsheim as my new neurologist.

Non-motor symptoms list can cause one to feel stressed. Are these symptoms part of the aging process? At this stage (seven years) issues appear the same.

Sleep has continued to be troublesome despite many of the suggestions made earlier in this report. I easily fall asleep but wake up at different times during the night. On awakening, my right side is quite stiff and usually take one Sinemet capsule to alleviate stiffness. Turning in bed is somewhat demanding at times. As usual, medications cause me to experience dreams throughout the night. Dreams are not negative, but silly in nature.

Cognitive skills remain focused. I appear to have lost some ability to smell. My taste does not appear to be affected. I've noticed a bit of weight loss, but this could be the result of constant workouts or aging.

April 3, 2014, Dr. Tamara Pringsheim Neurologist Report
- No cognitive impairment.
- Experiences occasional constipation and urinary frequency during daytime.
- No pronounced postural changes.
- There was no resting tremor in the office today. There was no dyskinesias.
- Barely detectable rigidity at the right elbow only. No evidence of bradykinesia in the upper or lower limbs.

- Gait revealed slight dystonic posturing of the right arm while walking.
- Altered medication slightly: one tablet of 100/25 mg Sinemet at 6 a.m., 10 a.m., 2 p.m., 6 p.m., 10 p.m.
- Take Mirapex 1.0 mg at 6 a.m., 2 p.m., 10 p.m.

VR's Reaction and Insights

As of April 30, 2014, I have been assigned to a new neurologist, Dr. Tamara Pringsheim. Dr. Pringsheim is an Assistant Professor with the Department of Clinical Neurosciences, Psychiatry, Paediatrics and Community Health Sciences, Faculty of Medicine, University of Calgary. She is Director of the Calgary Tourette and Paediatric Movement Disorder Clinic at the Alberta Children's Hospital. She also provides care for patients at the Movement Disorder Clinic at the Foothills Medical Centre. I am very pleased that she chose me to replace Dr. Suchowersky as my neurologist. She is knowledgeable, compassionate and attentive to my condition.

March 10, 2015, Dr. Pringsheim
- No evidence of hypomimia (a reduced degree of facial expression) or hypophonia (soft speech) and extra ocular (eyes or vision movements were full with normal blink rate).
- Mild bradykinesia more evident in his arms and legs, with some mild cogwheel rigidly on the right more than the left.
- Able to rise out of a chair without using his arms.
- Co-ordination was normal to finger-to-nose bilaterally.
- Gait assessment showed no shuffling, freezing, or end bloc turns, and he had a normal base.
- Voluntarily moving his arms, more to the right than left.
- Doing well 8 years into his diagnosis of presumed idiopathic Parkinson's disease.
- Suggested a prescription for Sinemet 100/25 mg five times daily (6:00, 9:00, 12 Noon, 4:00 pm, and 8:00 pm).

- Continue with Mirapex three times a day and warned him of potential side effects, including cognitive impairment, hallucinations, and impulse control disorder.

VR's Reaction and Insights

Dr. Pringsheim is very thorough in her examinations. She is most positive and provides excellent feedback regarding my symptoms. Often, she has a student do a preliminary examination before providing her own assessment. She is a good listener and very supportive of my condition. My appointments are scheduled for every six months. I feel fortunate in having Dr. Tamara Pringsheim as my neurologist.

Prior to my examination with Dr. Pringsheim, I stated that several changes occurred during 2017 that raised my level of anxiety. Most significantly, my older brother passed away two weeks prior to my clinic visit. I also had total right knee replacement on May 24, 2017. I've noticed that anxiety or low-level stress tends to increase the symptoms of PD.

March 21, 2017, Dr. Pringsheim
- The patient is relatively stable with no significant changes since our last visit.
- No neck rigidity to the right upper extremity.
- Minimal bradykinesia in his right hand with finger tapping, hand movements, and pronation or postural supination.
- Able to rise from a chair without difficulty.
- Normal gait length and blog turning and arm swing.
- A slightly stooped posture.
- Pull back test was negative.
- Discussion suggested that decreasing the total dose of pramipexole is necessary to prevent side effects as one gets older.
- Sinemet dose will remain the same. 100/25 mg five times daily
- Pramipexole will decrease by a half-tablet at night and will continue with 1 mg in the morning and noon.
- Vic finds that he is more anxious recently because of number of changes in his life.

- His brother passed away 2 weeks prior to clinic visit.
- He will undergo knee replacement in May 2027.
- Sleep appears less stressful.
- This 71-year-old gentlemen appears to be well controlled with current meds.
- We discussed decreasing pramipexole by one half a tablet a night.
- It was a pleasure being part of his care.

VR's Reaction and Insights

I was pleased that Dr. Pringsheim found little change in my symptoms since the last 6-month examination.

Three symptoms that have caused me the most concern. 1. Rigidity or stiffness occurring mostly in the early morning or evening. 2. Tremors occur mostly in the early morning or evening and intensify when I'm anxious. 3. Since the beginning, sleep disturbance has been a major issue. I wake up at three or four o'clock in the morning with a tremor on my right side. Sometimes I take one Sinemet tablet with some success. And yes, I have dreams.

I decided to state some goals of increasing my physical fitness through cardio and strength training. I like to travel, hike and play golf. I enjoy traveling two to three times a year. Another goal is being psychologically fit. I want to stay positive and enjoy life. I take guitar lessons and make every attempt to maintain normal routines.

September 19, 2017, Dr. Pringsheim
- Good motor control throughout the day.
- Appeared to be in good health.
- Experiences occasional tremor in his right arm and leg in late evening.
- No hallucinations or difficulties with cognition.
- No evidence of tremor during examination.
- No dyskinesia at rest.
- Tone was nearly normal bilaterally in the upper and lower limbs.
- Mild, barely detectable bradykinesia on the right side only.

- Gait examination was normal.
- No progression of the disease since our last examination.

VR's Reaction and Insights

At this point, the paper lists many motor and non-motor symptoms in sections, Part 1-4. Reading information on these symptom side effects is like trying to decipher a prescription warning.

As reported earlier, resting tremor, rigidity, and sleep disorder are major concerns.

I have no difficulty falling asleep but wake up every night around 3AM or 4 AM. My right side feels stiff and sometimes it is difficult to get back to sleep. Also, my right foot feels numb. There is little doubt that taking medication causes one to dream. Vivid dreams yes, but no hallucinations, just silly dreams.

Bladder and constipation are evident with PD. Frequency is a problem during the day, but not during the night.

Mobility is good during the day but becomes more challenging during late evenings.

Psoriasis (mainly scalp area) has been an annoyance for years and sometimes is enhanced by Parkinson's disease. My dermatologist sees me on a regular basis every six months keeping my health in check.

Dealing with Parkinson's disease raises the level of anxiety and tends to elevate symptoms.

As we age it is important to supplement with good vitamin add-ons, such as: Centrum Multi-Gummies for Adults, Jamieson B12, Webber Lutein Extra Strength (1 tablet daily/20 mg), and Life D3 (1 tablet daily/1000 IU).

Stiffness is very noticeable either early morning or late at night. I work out at the Crowfoot YMCA four to five times a week. Exercise is very important to relieve stiffness. I begin workouts at 7 AM for about one and one-half hours. I enjoy the social aspect working out with the same people currently. I mix workout routines to stay motivated. To warm up, I use the stationary bike or treadmill for 20-30 minutes.

March 6, 2018, Dr. Pringsheim
- Vic was alert and appropriate throughout the examination.
- On cranial nerve examination, pupils were equal and reactive to light.
- No RAPD.
- Fundoscopy (examining the inside of the eye) was normal.
- Visual acuity and fields were normal. Extra-ocular movements were full.
- Facial sensation and muscle movements were symmetric.
- Palate and tongue were midline.
- Hearing was grossly normal.
- Sternocleidomastoid (muscles that control the neck) and trap strength were full.
- Tongue strength was full.
- On motor examination, he had normal bulk, tone, and strength.
- He did have a mild resting tremor in his right hand with distraction.
- Mild bradykinesia in his upper and lower extremity.
- Reflexes were 2+ throughout with downing toes.
- Sensation was grossly normal to temperature and touch.
- Finger to nose was grossly (extremely) normal with some mild tremor his right hand.
- On gait examination, he had a slight abnormal movement of his right arm but was otherwise normal.
- On Romberg he had mild drift backwards.
- No significant changes at this time, however continue our slow wean off the pramipexole.
- Continue Sinemet 100/25 mg 6 times per day. Decrease pramipexole to 1 mg b.i.d.
- Contact us should he have any questions and concerns sooner.

VR's Reaction and Insights

2017 has been quite the challenge. It began with a torn ligament in my right hand because I fell up the basement stairs trying to carry two wine bottles. Nothing broke but my finger hurt.

My major challenge was the replacement of my right knee. I was unable to do much cardio strength training during the summer months, except basic exercise routines. Since my knee operation, I made the effort to improve my cardio strength training to slow down the progression of Parkinson's disease.

In addition, I had to deal with a minor operation for sun damage, a touch of arthritis in my left hand and a change in my family doctor.

As of November, I finally gave up teaching at the university. I wasn't unhappy to kiss 2017 goodbye.

This past year has been a significant challenge to reach this goal. I want to maintain a positive attitude of life and not worry about the mind anxiety experienced in 2017.

October 11, 2018, Dr. Pringsheim
- The patient appears well with a resting tremor affecting his jaw and right side (high amplitude and low frequency tremor).
- Memory is good and does not experience hallucinations.
- Mild rigidity on right side as well as bradykinesia.
- Examined feet and did not find any convincing sensory defects in either lower limb.
- Continue to withdraw Mirapex to 0.5 mg three times daily.
- Increasing levodopa to 1 1/2 mg five times daily.
- Medication prescribed Sinemet 100/25 mg one tablet five times daily and Mirapex 1 mg and 0.5 mg in the afternoon and evening
- Encouraged him to try reading/practicing mindfulness for his anxiety.
- Reassured the patient that he is doing well.

VR's Reaction and Insights

What am I experiencing since my last examination on October 11, 2018?

I have noted slight progression of the disease. Both resting tremor and rigidity remain main concerns. Resting tremor is more noticeable when feeling anxious. When travelling and on vacation, the symptoms appear less of a problem. Rigidity is more evident in my trunk (lower back and buttocks) area, especially in early morning. On occasion, my right knee feels stiff and right foot feels numb.

Sometimes medication takes 15-20 minutes to take effect and lasts for about 3 1/2 hours. I am not experiencing any dyskinesias or difficulty with my gait. General mood is good and described as upbeat. I have not experienced any falls to date and no memory or cognitive issues. I find it difficult to fall into a deep sleep, but the clonazepam does help suppress vivid dreams. I continue to remain active exercising 4-5 times per week. To sharpen my cognitive skills, I attempt to play guitar, electric keyboard and golf. I've also decided to increase my walking outdoors on a regular schedule.

April 30, 2019, Dr. Pringsheim
- On physical examination, the patient appeared well.
- There was a resting tremor affecting the right upper limb.
- No dyskinesias at rest or provoked through examination.
- Very mild rigidity bilaterally and minimal bradykinesia of all four limbs.
- Gait was normal.
- Suggested getting mild anxiety under control as it seems to have an impact on his motor symptoms.
- Recommended that he try mindfulness-based cognitive theory for his anxiety.
- Might try cannabis oil as another solution.
- Currently taking Sinemet 100/25 mg 1 1/2 tablets five times daily, Mirapex 0.5 mg three times daily, and clonazepam 0.5 mg at bedtime.

VR's Reaction and Insights

My next visit and examination with Dr. Pringsheim will be scheduled October 29, 2019. Unfortunately, I received a letter during the summer that Dr. Pringsheim has taken a leave of absence because of illness. It is hoped that she will return to the clinic as her condition improves.

Dr. Sarah Furtado has graciously accepted to be her replacement until she returns. I am scheduled to meet with Dr Furtado on Tuesday, October 29, 2019, at 9:00 A.M. in Health Science Centre, 1st Floor Area 3.

October 29, 2019, Dr. Sarah Furtado, Neurologist Report
- The patient has a remarkable history dating back to January 19, 2007.
- He continues Sinemet regular 100/25 mg, 1 1/2 tablets each at 5:00, 9:00, AM 12:00 Noon, 4:00, and 8:00 PM
- Also, Mirapex 0.25 mg two tablets each at 9:00 AM, 12:00 PM and 4:00 PM.
- At bedtime, he may choose to take 0.5 clonazepam or administer 5 gm of Melatonin to help him with a regular sleep pattern.
- He admits suggested times become disjointed when busy working on different projects.
- Medications kick in within 15-20 minutes and sometimes wear off before the next scheduled dosage.
- He does not have dyskinesias, but experiences resting tremor during wear off times.
- He has no postural hypotension, no hallucinations, and no confusion.
- A rested sleep continues to be bothersome waking up around 3:00 AM.
- On examination, I noticed a slight diminishment in facial expression and voice volume.
- No resting tremor, but mild bradykinesia.
- No dyskinesias, good stride length and arm swing.
- During this hour and one-half examination, I reinforced that he is doing quite well.
- I emphasized him to try taking medications on a more regular basis.
- I renewed his medications and will see him in six months' time.

VR's Reaction and Insights

As of January 19, 2020, I will have dealt with Parkinson's disease for 13 years. I must admit to being anxious having to be examined by a new neurologist substituting for Dr. Pringsheim.

The question remains: "What motor and non-motor symptoms continue to appear troublesome up to January 2020?" Rigidity and resting tremor are the main culprits. Rigidity is more evident in the trunk region (lower back and buttocks) area. Resting tremor is more evident when tired or getting out of bed in the early morning. Normal sleep patterns are disrupted because of lack of medication while sleeping.

Dr. Furtado suggested chewing on one tablet of Sinemet may help return to a more normal sleep pattern. I should also mention that my meeting and examination with Dr. Furtado was extremely positive as she showed a caring and professional interest in my condition. I would imagine feeling fortunate that many of the other PD symptoms are either mild or non-existent.

Cognitive skills remained focused. I am not experiencing any dyskinesias or difficulty with my gait. Overall, my general mood is good and described as up-beat. I will admit to a slight progression of overall symptoms which sometimes causes anxiety. I am also aware that my central nervous system is much more sensitive as the result of PD disease. Anxiety can intensify my over-all condition.

I continue to remain active exercising 4-5 times per week at the local YMCA. To sharpen my cognitive skills, I attempt to play guitar and piano. During the summer, I play golf on a more regular basis. This winter, I hope to ski and skate as a means of increasing my exercise.

March 11, 2020, Global Pandemic. A Significant Date
Why is this date significant? March 11, 2020, introduced an infectious disease called Coronavirus disease (COVID-19) and caused a global pandemic around the World.

Most people infected with the virus would experience mild to moderate respiratory illness and recover without requiring special treatment. However, some would become seriously ill and require medical attention. Older people and those with underlying medical conditions like cardiovascular disease, diabetes, chronic respiratory disease, or cancer were more likely to develop serious illness. Anyone could get sick with COVID-19 and become seriously ill or die at any age. Fortunately, I remained healthy and was not infected by the virus.

November 26, 2020, Dr. Pringsheim
- Zoom was used as a platform in lieu of meeting at the regular hospital location because of CoVid-19.
- Conversation centered around the "anxiety" symptom as related to PD.
- Stressed the importance of cutting back on alcohol as a means of relieving anxiety.
- Suggested one-half glass of wine a day or limited to special occasions only.
- Other means to control anxiety is practicing "mindfulness" and through exercising.
- Taking 0.5 mg of lorazepam as needed under your tongue and make your anxiety more manageable.

VR's Reaction and Insights

Found it strange to use Zoom as a platform for discussion. Talked about anxiety brought on by the Global Pandemic and CoVid-19. Was aware that anxiety can result when medication is less effective during "off periods. Mentioned that a glass of wine at dinner time helps to relax the body. Agreed that too much alcohol will bring out the symptoms more, especially during off-times. One-half a glass of wine is permissible and special occasions. Practicing "mindfulness" is difficult because I tend to fall asleep. Continue exercising on a regular basis.

July 6, 2021, Dr. Pringsheim
- The patient makes my job easy with his outlines and questions completed before each appointment.
- How are you feeling overall? Are you ever frozen or stuck?
- How are you sleeping?
- Do you ever have hallucinations? Any falls?

- Have you practiced mindfulness?
- Do you feel fear about your future?
- Any problems with urination?
- Do you understand the therapeutic window? The therapeutic window is a narrowing of the gap between "off and on" times.
- When your body tends to wiggle you are at the end of your dosage...starting up you feel more tremor.
- We will continue to decrease your Mirapex as part of a slow process.
- The patient is hard on himself...somewhat of a perfectionist.
- As requested, his appointments will be scheduled for mornings.
- I haven't seen his for two years because of my personal leave of absence. His appearance and PD symptoms show little change.

VR's Reaction and Insights

Generally, feeling OK.... challenging time before supper or specifically during off times. I take my meds every 3.5 hours between dosages. I try my best to understand terms such as wearing off effect, and the struggle with on-off phenomena. Essentially, what I think is meant is that over-time, the positive effect of medication simply wears off before the next dose. I may experience heightened symptoms of PD disease. The usual solution is to shorten the time between doses.

Phenomena which is unique to Parkinson's disease refers to PWP ability to perform common physical activities one minute and then be totally incapable. I should try to track my own off fluctuations and then report my findings to my neurologist. Is there a reoccurring pattern? Sleep issues have been a major problem since I was diagnosed. Over time, sleep issues have somewhat improved. I do not hallucinate.

You asked about COVID because it caused anxiety for most people. Lately, life has become somewhat normal. We see the family on a regular basis for dinners and special occasions. I have all my shots to date.

Urination is not affected but becomes a somewhat nuisance during daytime frequencies. Practicing mindfulness doesn't appear to lower anxiety. I tend to fall asleep. I appreciate your suggestion trying it again in a less comfortable position. Ironically, I experience anxiety doing the research on my PD Manuscript.

I am successful at performing various exercises asked by Dr. Pringsheim, such as getting up from a chair without aids; tapping my feet; flexing my hands; and walking down the corridor emphasizing my gait.

Meds remain the same between 9 to 10 tablets a day. I can be flexible taking an extra tablet when needed.

October 25, 2022, Dr. Pringsheim

- Dr. Pringsheim asked the patient what symptoms he was experiencing since our last meeting.
- Sighs indicate that he is doing well. He can maintain all tasks around the house. He keeps himself active by exercising on a regular basis at the YMCA. He plays golf in the spring and summer.
- I tested his coordination and balance while observing his walk, stance, sit, turn, extend my arms and hands, and so on.
- He stated that he was somewhat anxious due to the Global Pandemic, his brother's death, and was told by his family doctor that he was leaving the profession.
- I reinforced that anxiety is quite normal. Especially, if a person is diagnosed with a chronic disease.
- In his case his anxiety is quite normal considering the circumstances.

VR's Reaction and Insights

Symptoms are what you tell your neurologist as opposed to signs what your neurologist observes during the examination. I was pleased that her observations were positive. Again, she emphasized that I was doing well, and few could tell I had Parkinson's disease. I talked about loss of weight (5 pounds). She said that it is normal as one ages. I mentioned that I was examined by a doctor at Group 23 at Canada Olympic Park to check my knee replacement. He would see me again in April 2023. I've tried to increase my range of motion so that I can ski and make use of my bicycle.

The last two and one-half years have been stressful because of the Global Pandemic and Covid-19. My brother passed away at the start of Covid-19. Sad to say that my family doctor has decided to leave the profession. Finding a new doctor has been a stressful task. I asked my neurologist whether the drug called clonazepam 0.5 mg taken every night is addictive.

May 16, 2023, Dr. Pringsheim
- Dr. Pringsheim asked about current medications.
- Confirming lava-dopa five times a day., pramipexole .375 mg twice a day and Clonazepam at bedtime.
- Vic found a new doctor who has a very good reputation.
- He's feeling a little more stiffness and more tremor in his right side.
- Sometimes he forgets to take his medications when he is busy. Uses a dose set box to keep track of them.
- Wearing off time is much the same as before about 3 1/2 hours.
- Increased anxiety due to continuing to write his book about Parkinson's. He stated that it is nearly finished.
- Managing his anxiety by taking breaks and doing something else.
- Still goes to the YMCA, takes walks is playing some games with family.
- No difficulties with memory, no hallucinations or delusions, or with impulse control
- Hasn't had a dose failure.
- Not shuffling his feet except in early morning. Body is stiff when he gets up. Is careful about going down the stairs.
- Tense in the right arm but other tests are fine.
- Sometimes dizzy when anxious or tired
- We talked about new treatment coming out next year - a sub-cutaneous lava-dopa injection.

VR's Reaction and Insights

There is no change in my medications. I'm pleased. When Dr. Leaman left I was able to find a doctor the name of Dr. S. Raj. My neurologist knows of her and states that she has a good reputation. I've been feeling more anxiety of late probably due to writing this manuscript. I've learned a lot about Parkinson's in doing my research.

I sincerely hope that others will benefit reading this manuscript and choosing their own right road in helping others.

APPENDIX 2:
Rating Symptoms

PARKINSON RATING SYMPTOMS ASSESSMENT

This chart is designed to give a quick assessment of the various motor and non-motor symptoms of Parkinson's disease as they affect me personally.

VR Peterson
As of August 2023

MOTOR SYMPTOMS	RARELY NOTICEABLE	MILDLY NOTICEABLE	MORE NOTICEABLE	EXTREMELY NOTICEABLE
Resting Tremor			✓	
Rigidity			✓	
Bradykinesia	✓			
Balance Problems	✓			

NON-MOTOR SYMPTOMS	RARELY NOTICEABLE	MILDLY NOTICEABLE	MORE NOTICEABLE	EXTREMELY NOTICEABLE
Dyskinesia		✓		
Side Effects		✓		
Behaviour	✓			
Stress		✓		
Anxiety		✓		
Hallucinations Delusions	✓			
Mobility		✓		
Vision	✓			
Speech		✓		
Effect on Blood Pressure		✓		
Sleep Problems (Insomnia)		✓		
Effect on Skin		✓		
Effect on Sex Life		✓		

NON-MOTOR SYMPTOMS	RARELY NOTICEABLE	MILDLY NOTICEABLE	MORE NOTICEABLE	EXTREMELY NOTICEABLE
Constipation and bowel problems		✓		
Bladder problems		✓		
Feeling faint		✓		
Leg swelling	✓			
Pain	✓			
Double vision		✓		
Cognitive Impairment	✓			
Changes in taste and smell		✓		
Unexplained changes in weight		✓		

APPENDIX 3:
Glossary

1   **Dopamine** – A chemical released in the brain that makes you feel good. It is a type of neurotransmitter.

2   **Dopamine agonist** – a drug that activates certain types of cells called dopamine receptors.

3   **Bradykinesia** – means slowness of movement and is one of the cardinal manifestations of Parkinson's disease. Weakness, tremor and rigidity may contribute to but not fully explain bradykinesia.

4   **Amantadine** – a drug that is used to treat Parkinson's and its symptoms including dyskinesia (uncontrolled movements).

5   **Trazadone** – a medication used to treat depression and help patients with sleep problems.

6   **Domperidone** – a drug used to treat nausea and vomiting caused by other drugs.

7   **Omeprazole** – used to treat certain conditions where there is too much acid in the stomach.

8   **Apo-Levocarb 100/25mg** – **a** drug used to treat Parkinson's disease. Levodopa is converted to dopamine in the brain. It comes in regular pills or CR controlled release pills.

9   **Pms-Clonazepam .05mg** – a drug that belongs to the benzodiazepine family. It is used to reduce anxiety or to help induce sleep.

10   **Sinemet** – a widely prescribed drug used to treat Parkinson's disease. It is often considered the gold standard for Parkinson's treatment. It's two main active ingredients are carbidopa and levodopa. Levodopa is converted to dopamine in the brain.

11   **Substantia nigra** – is a critical brain region for the production of dopamine. It is part of your basal ganglia and is essential in how your brain controls your body movements/. It also plays a part in the chemical signalling in your brain, which affects learning, mood, judgement, decision-making and other processes.

12   **Deep Brain Stimulation (DBS)** – is an elective surgical procedure in which electrodes are implanted into certain brain areas. These

electrodes, or leads, generate electrical impulses that control abnormal brain activity.

13   **Double Blinded Placebo Control Trial** – is where both the subjects and the researchers do not know who is getting the drug or the placebo.

14   **Dyskinesias** – are voluntary, erratic, writhing movements of the face, arms, legs or trunk.

15   **Melatonin** – is a hormone that your brain produces in response to darkness. It helps with the timing of your circadian rhythms (24-hour internal clock) and with sleep. '

16   **Serotonin** – is a chemical that carries messages between nerve cells in the brain and throughout your body.

17   **Pramipexole** – is a dopamine agonist that works on the nervous system to help treat the symptoms of Parkinson's disease. I am taking Auro-Pramipexole 0.75 mg or Mirapex.

18   **SLV308** – is the drug used in the first trial in which I participated. It is the drug's only identifier.

19   **Creatine** – is ana amino acid located mostly in your body's muscles as well as in the brain.

20   **UPDRS** – Unified Parkinson's Disease Rating Scale has four parts. Each part has multiple points that are individually scored using zero for normal or no problems, one for minimal problems, two for mild problems, three for moderate problems and four for severs problems.

Acknowledgements

Tamara Pringsheim, MD, Assistant Professor, Department of Clinical Neurosciences, Faculty of. Medicine, University of Calgary. Dr. Pringsheim is my personal neurologist playing the lead in my journey against PD.

Oksana Suchowersky, MD, FRCPC, University of Calgary Medical Clinic. Dr. Suchowersky diagnosed my disease providing excellent care during the initial stages of PD.

McCabe, P. Kevin MD, General Practitioner, Valley Ridge Medical Centre (Retired) Dr. McCabe was my GP until he retired as my GP in 2018.

Leaman, Todd MD, General Practitioner, Valley Ridge Medical Center (Retired). Dr. Leaman was my GP until he retired as my GP in September 2022.

References

Argue, John Parkinson's Disease The Art of Moving. Oakland CA: New Harbinger Publications Inc., 2000.

Bauer-Wu, Susan, PHD, RN. Leaves Falling Gently, Oakland, CA: New Harbinger Publications, Inc. 2011.

Bourne, Edmund. Anxiety & Phobia Workbook: Fourth Edition, Oakland, CA: New Harbinger Publications, Inc. 2005.

Fox, Michael J. Always Looking Up: The Adventures of An Incurable Optimist, New York: Hyperion, 2009.

Marie, Lianna. Everything You Wanted to Know About Parkinson's Disease, 2015.

Palfreman, Jon. Brain Storms: Parkinson's and the Race to Unlock the Secrets of One of the Brain's Most Mysterious Diseases. Toronto, Canada: Harper Collins Publishing, Ltd. 2015.

Postuma, Ronald, MD, MSc. Julius Anang, MD Parkinson's Disease: An Introductory Guide, McGill University Health Centre, 2nd Edition, 2017.

Tagliati, Michele, MD; Gary N. Guten, MD, MA; and Jo Horne, MA. "Parkinson's Disease for Dummies," 2007.